Praise for JORGE CRUISE
from Doctors and Experts

"Stubborn Fat Gone!™ *is jam-packed with good science and good sense. This program is fabulous!"*

— CHRISTIANE NORTHUP, M.D.,
Ob-gyn and author of the *New York Times* bestsellers
Women's Bodies, Women's Wisdom and *The Wisdom of Menopause*

"Thanks, Jorge . . . for always Walking the Walk!"

— LESLIE SANSONE,
Creator of the Walk at Home workouts

"When it comes to your health, forward thinking will allow you to avoid obesity and disease and achieve longevity. Jorge's program springs from progressive science that can truly change your body."

— RAY KURZWEIL,
World-renowned scientist and author of *The Singularity Is Near: When Humans Transcend Biology* and *Fantastic Voyage: Live Long Enough to Live Forever*

"Jorge, again, is on to something; belly fat is surely an indicator of poor health."

— SUZANNE SOMERS,
Actress and best-selling author of *Breakthrough: Eight Steps to Wellness*

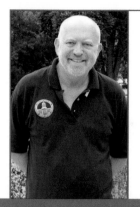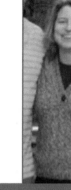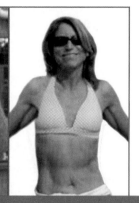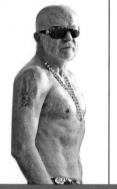

Ken lost 60 lbs.   Amy lost 40 lbs.

"No matter how much or how little weight you want to lose, you absolutely can do it if you just believe in yourself!" — Anthony

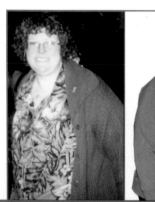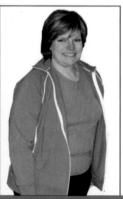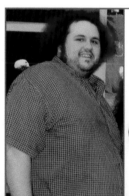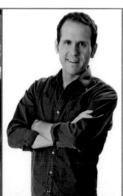

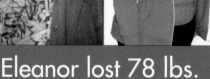

Eleanor lost 78 lbs.   Anthony lost 210 lbs.

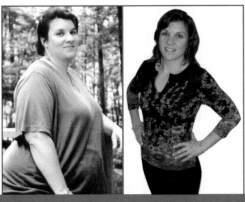

Maria lost 155 lbs.

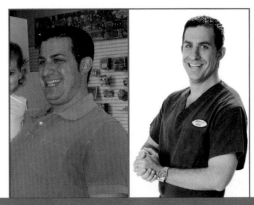

Jon lost 40 lbs.

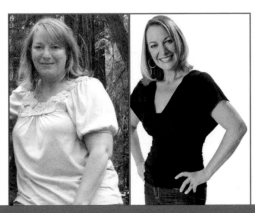

Amber lost 54 lbs.

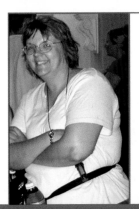

Michelle lost 86 lbs.

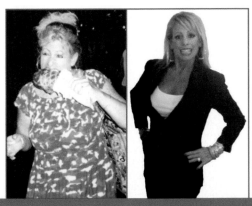

Kelly lost 68 lbs.

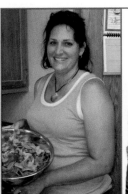
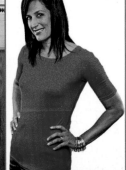

Kelli lost 30 lbs.

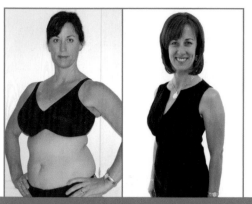

Michelle lost 20 lbs.

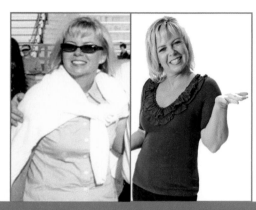

Darla lost 25 lbs.

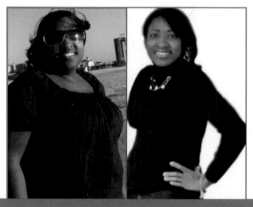

Ashlee lost 92 lbs.

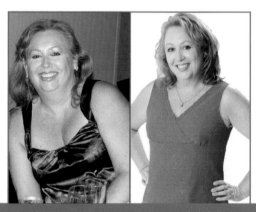

Deborah lost 72 lbs.

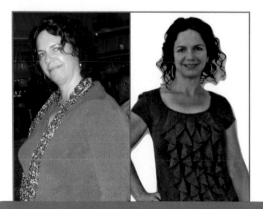

Rosalie lost 85 lbs.

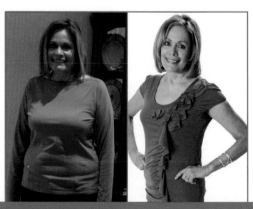

Gloria lost 20 lbs.

"All you have to do is believe in yourself and follow Jorge's recommendations, and everything else will fall back into place." — Darla

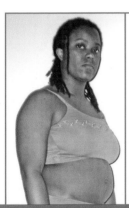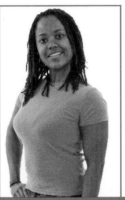

Alexandra lost 16 lbs.

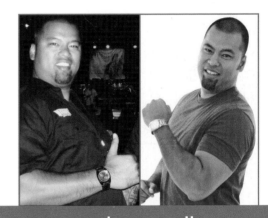

Ron lost 20 lbs.

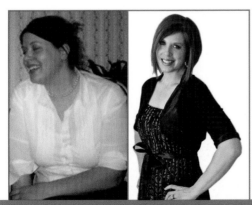

Ashley lost 50 lbs.

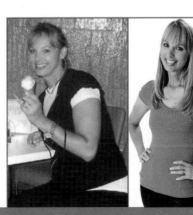

Alicia lost 15 lbs.

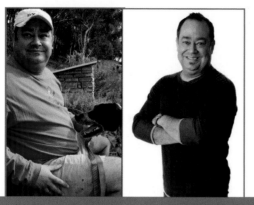

Karl lost 35 lbs.

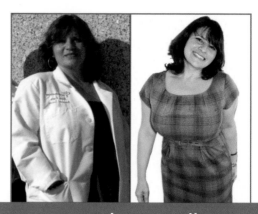

Maria lost 30 lbs.

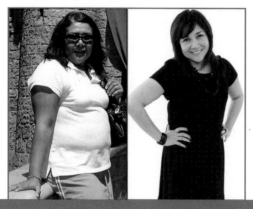

Mirian lost 42 lbs.

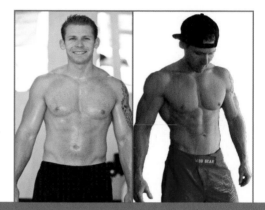

Stephen lost 13 lbs.

"I gave Jorge's plan a shot and I've finally found what truly works." — Nicole

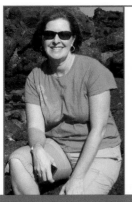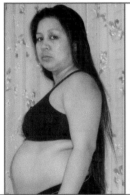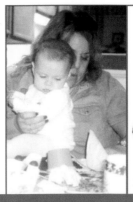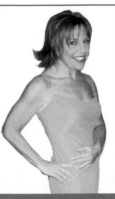

Robin lost 40 lbs.

Nancy lost 115 lbs.

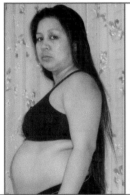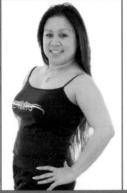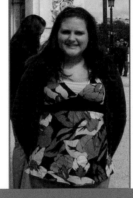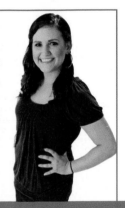

Karen lost 16 lbs.

Jessica lost 58 lbs.

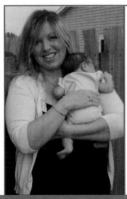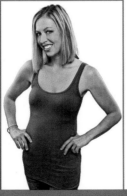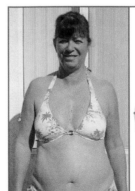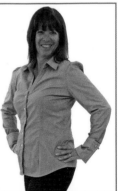

Nicole lost 86 lbs.

Kim lost 18 lbs.

stubborn fat gone!™

Other Books by
JORGE CRUISE

Happy Hormones, Slim Belly™

The 100™

Inches Off™

The Aging Cure™

The Belly Fat Cure™

The Belly Fat Cure™ *Sugar & Carb Counter*

The Belly Fat Cure™ *Fast Track*

The Belly Fat Cure™ *Quick Meals*

The Belly Fat Cure™ *Diet*

Body at Home™

The 12-Second Sequence™

The 12-Second Sequence™ *Journal*

The 3-Hour Diet™

The 3-Hour Diet™ *Cookbook*

The 3-Hour Diet™ *for Teens*

The 3-Hour Diet™ *On-the-Go*

8 Minutes in the Morning®

8 Minutes in the Morning® *for Extra-Easy Weight Loss*

8 Minutes in the Morning® *for a Perfect Body*

8 Minutes in the Morning® *for Real Shapes, Real Sizes*

8 Minutes in the Morning® *to a Flat Belly*

8 Minutes in the Morning® *to Lean Hips and Thin Thighs*

PLEASE VISIT:

Hay House USA: www.hayhouse.com®
Hay House Australia: www.hayhouse.com.au
Hay House UK: www.hayhouse.co.uk
Hay House South Africa: www.hayhouse.co.za
Hay House India: www.hayhouse.co.in

stubborn
fat
gone!™

discover Think Fit™ to turn off
stress and lose 1.5 lbs. every day

jorge cruise

HAY
HOUSE

HAY HOUSE, INC.
Carlsbad, California • New York City
London • Sydney • Johannesburg
Vancouver • Hong Kong • New Delhi

Published and distributed in the United States by: Hay House, Inc.: www.hayhouse.com® • *Published and distributed in Australia by:* Hay House Australia Pty. Ltd.: www.hayhouse.com.au • *Published and distributed in the United Kingdom by:* Hay House UK, Ltd.: www.hayhouse.co.uk • *Published and distributed in the Republic of South Africa by:* Hay House SA (Pty), Ltd.: www.hayhouse.co.za • *Distributed in Canada by:* Raincoast Books: www.raincoast.com • *Published in India by:* Hay House Publishers India: www.hayhouse.co.in

The JorgeCruise.com, Inc., team: *Managing director:* Oliver Stephenson/JorgeCruise.com, Inc. • *Executive assistant:* Kristin Penne/JorgeCruise.com, Inc.

Notice: The information given here is designed to help you make informed decisions about your body and health. The suggestions for specific foods in this program are not intended to replace appropriate or necessary medical care. Before starting any diet or exercise program, always see your physician. If you have specific medical symptoms, consult your physician immediately. If any recommendations given in this program contradict your physician's advice, be sure to consult him or her before proceeding. Mention of specific products, companies, organizations, or authorities in this book does not imply endorsement by the author or the publisher; nor does mention of specific companies, organizations, or authorities in the book imply that they endorse this book. The author and the publisher disclaim any liability or loss, personal or otherwise, resulting from the procedures in this program.

Product pictures, trademarks, and trademark names are used throughout this book to describe and inform the reader about various proprietary products that are owned by others. The presentation of such information is intended to benefit the owner of the products and trademarks and is not intended to infringe upon trademark, copyright, or other rights; nor to imply any claim to the mark other than that made by the owner. No endorsement of the information contained in this book has been given by the owners of such products and trademarks, and no such endorsement is implied by the inclusion of product trademarks in this book.

The reference material in this book was compiled using a number of sources, and all information was accurate at the time of printing. Internet addresses given in this book were accurate at the time the book went to press.

TRADEMARKS

The Belly Fat Cure	8 Minutes in the Morning	Stubborn Fat Gone
S/C Value	Happy Hormones, Slim Belly	The 100
Carb Swap System	3-Hour Diet	Women's Carb Cycling
Sugar Calories	Skinny Waffle	Think Fit
Eat Fit	Simply Fit	Move Fit

Library of Congress Control Number: 2014957611

ISBN: 978-1-4019-4722-4

10 9 8 7 6 5 4 3 2 1
1st edition, April 2015

PRINTED IN THE UNITED STATES OF AMERICA

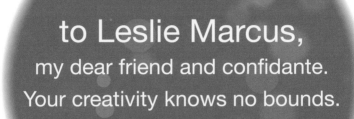

to Leslie Marcus,
my dear friend and confidante.
Your creativity knows no bounds.

contents

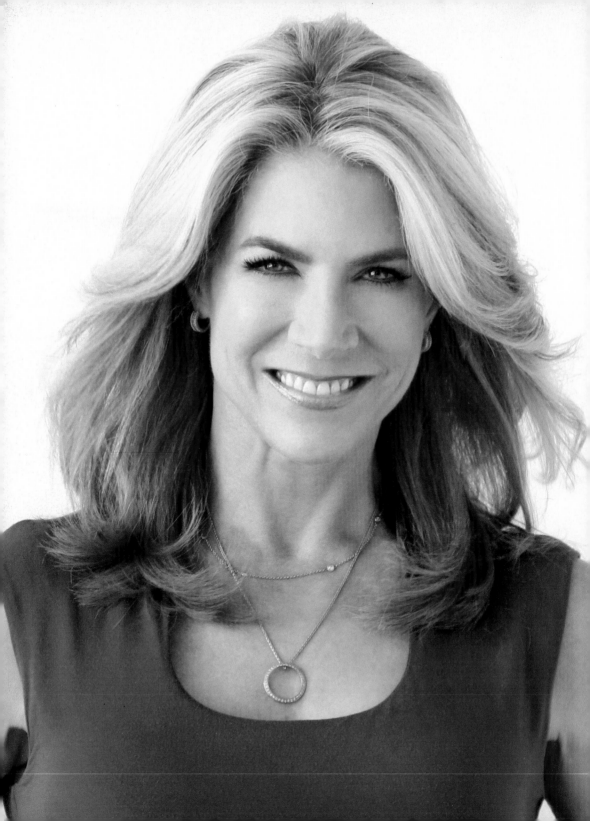

foreword

Jorge Cruise has designed an intelligent, easy-to-implement plan that helps you once and for all ditch stubborn belly fat. He understands that you want fast results and don't have hours to prepare elaborate recipes or work out at the gym. Simplicity is key here, and he breaks it down into three easy components: Think Fit™, Eat Fit™, and Move Fit™.

Jorge removes the guesswork at each step of the plan. As you read, it is just like having him at your side, guiding and encouraging you every day.

Over the next 12 weeks, you will become more mindful of your choices and your thoughts. I strongly suggest that you track your success with journaling. Writing everything down will reinforce your new eating, exercise, and thinking habits. Practicing daily affirmations will create an optimistic mind-set to help you stay the course.

How you do one thing determines how you do everything. You might begin this program wanting to lose stubborn belly fat (and you will), but along the way you'll reduce your risk for disease, feel and look better, and find a new vitality and zeal.

That's why *Stubborn Fat Gone!*™ ultimately transcends being a diet book to become something much more personal. Fat loss becomes a metaphor for life: Succeed here and everything improves.

Enjoy the journey!

— JJ VIRGIN, CNS, CHFS,

Celebrity nutrition and fitness expert JJ Virgin helps clients lose weight fast by breaking free from food intolerances and crushing their sugar cravings. She is the author of the *New York Times* bestsellers *The Virgin Diet: Drop 7 Foods, Lose 7 Pounds, Just 7 Days*; *The Virgin Diet Cookbook: 150 Easy and Delicious Recipes to Lose Weight and Feel Better Fast*; and *JJ Virgin's Sugar Impact Diet: Drop 7 Hidden Sugars, Lose up to 10 Pounds in Just 2 Weeks*. JJ is also a frequent blogger at *The Huffington Post*, MindBodyGreen, and other outlets as well as a popular guest on TV, radio, and in magazines. Learn more at www.jjvirgin.com.

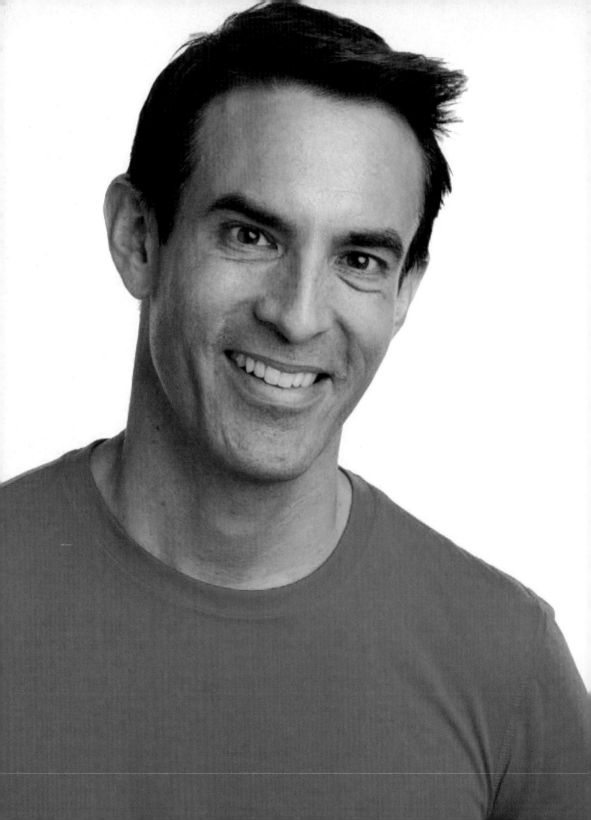

welcome to **Stubborn Fat Gone!**™

For over a decade my passion has been focused on helping millions achieve health and lose weight, specifically targeting the fat that bothers them most—**BELLY FAT.** It can ruin a trip to the beach, a night out on the town, or a simple school function. For many, it may seem that no matter what programs they try or what trendy diet they're doing, that dangerous, stubborn fat just won't go away, leaving them more frustrated and stressed out.

This is my first book ever to focus on the hidden component that affects your weight . . . **stress.** When your stress hormones are activated, it triggers your body to produce more belly fat. I have learned, after working with so many of my online and celebrity clients who are eating a diet low in Sugar Calories, that stubborn belly fat will not come off unless you have control over your stress hormones.

Stubborn Fat Gone™ is a brand-new plan that goes beyond telling you the foods to eat to lose 1.5 lbs. a day and finally addresses this missing component that has kept you frustrated for so long. I call this stress-free approach to boosting your mind-set Think Fit™.

This book combines the best science along with the newest research on losing the most difficult fat in a complete 12-week plan. Think of this book as your lifestyle makeover with me as your personal coach for each step of the way. Before you start, I also suggest that you go to Facebook.com/JorgeCruise and join my fan page to meet other people on this plan and get additional support.

I am excited to be part of your journey and see your full transformation!

Your coach,

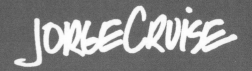

01

the frustration of stubborn belly fat

It's not your fault.

Every day, while I'm working with clients on my Facebook page, all I hear is how difficult it is to get rid of belly fat. It's a familiar struggle. Back when John F. Kennedy took office and Martin Luther King, Jr., proclaimed "I have a dream," over 2 million Americans were obese (13 percent of the population). Today the number stands at 35 percent of the population, nearly 110 million Americans. When you include those who are *overweight*, that number swells dramatically. According to the National Health and Nutrition Examination Survey, two-thirds of Americans (more than 215 million people) are now overweight or obese.

Perhaps even more sobering is the fact that in all that time, we've been trying so hard to lose weight. According to recent statistics, approximately 108 million Americans are currently dieting. People are counting calories, pumping iron, and visiting surgeons, all in a desperate attempt to shed pounds. Despite the fact that we spent $60.5 *billion* in 2013 on weight loss, our waistlines continue to expand, rather than shrink. As much money as we spend as a nation, the obesity epidemic just won't go away.

On the covers of celebrity magazines like *People, Closer,* and *Us Weekly,* headlines are always touting how some celebrity stays slim with the latest dieting trend and promising to

The Dangers of Belly Fat

Belly fat is a leading contributor to many of the top health concerns in America. Having an excess of even 2 percent more belly fat than average comes with a 39 percent increased risk of developing one of the following:

- heart disease
- type 2 diabetes
- cancer
- heart attack

show us how we too can work off the pounds. We wonder if we could lose the weight if only we had the "right" genetics, expensive personal training, steel-like willpower, and the best surgeons money could buy. But what if I told you that it was simpler than all that?

Are You Feeling Stressed?

More than just poor dieting or exercise habits, the hidden component affecting our weight is **stress that activates our stress hormones.** It's so insidious and so prevalent in our lives that the American Psychological Association (APA) calls chronic stress "a public health crisis." According to the APA's recent Stress in America survey, 22 percent of Americans reported being under severe stress, and 44 percent reported that their stress levels have increased in the past five years.

There are two categories of stress: distress and eustress. Most people recognize that negative life events cause stress, such as getting divorced, losing a loved one, having a difficult job, or struggling to pay bills. This is "distress," which results from unpleasant situations. But what a lot of people don't realize is that happy events can be stressful, too. Getting married, having a baby, meeting new people, working at a rewarding job, or any other positive experience that causes you to feel motivated and excited causes "eustress." The common denominator is change. Really, *any* change is stressful.

Stress Equals Belly Fat

When you're stressed, your hypothalamus, a tiny region at the base of your forebrain, sends a signal to your pituitary gland that prompts your adrenal glands, located atop your kidneys, to release a surge of hormones, mainly the stress hormone cortisol. It doesn't matter whether you're rushing to meet a deadline or running away from a hungry lion, your body's response is the same: release cortisol to keep your blood sugar up and give you the energy you need to deal with the stressor.

At the proper level in your body, cortisol helps maintain blood pressure and blood sugar levels, acts as an anti-inflammatory, and helps regulate the immune system. Really, it acts as a protective mechanism for your body. It also helps you mobilize fat from storage to be used as energy. When in check, cortisol is a wonderful aid for your health.

However, your system is not equipped to deal with consistently high levels of this hormone. Going back to our example, if you were worried about becoming lion lunch, once you escaped, your body would calm and your cortisol levels would go down as well. But these days, there's always a deadline— or a bill, or a relationship challenge, or a thousand messages to reply to. It seems like you can never escape the stress, so your cortisol levels are chronically high, building up in your blood and wreaking havoc in a number of ways. A study published in the journal *Obesity Research* found that when overweight women were exposed to stress for an hour, those who had a high waist-to-hip ratio (and therefore more abdominal fat) secreted more cortisol than those who had a low ratio. When the researchers delved into their backgrounds, they discovered that the women with bigger waists had poorer coping skills and more mood swings.

What a lot of people don't realize is that happy events can be stressful, too.

While all of the women in the study became angry in response to the stressful tasks they were given, what's interesting is that the women with bigger waists showed less anger. The scientists speculated that was because these women felt helpless in the face of the stress. They suggested that a person's coping strategy might influence how her body reacts to stress, releases cortisol, and distributes fat. Stress combined with more coping skills equals more fat.

Another study, this one conducted at Yale University, found that stress was linked to excess abdominal fat even in otherwise slender women. The researchers exposed women to stressful situations over a period of four days. The women with greater waist-to-hip ratios, whether they were overweight or slim, felt more threatened, performed worse on the tests, and secreted more cortisol. Even during the later days, the slim women with high waist-to-hip ratios secreted more cortisol in response to the laboratory stress than the slim women with low ratios. **The scientists concluded that having more belly fat makes you more vulnerable to stress.**

Another factor in weight gain is that high cortisol levels increase appetite and cravings. A study published in the journal *Appetite* found that when people were under chronic stress, they were hungrier, felt more cravings for non-nutritious foods, and struggled with disinhibited eating and bingeing. Unfortunately, when we're stressed, we tend to reach for poor choices rather than a grilled chicken salad.

Stress and Belly Fat Are Killing Us

Elevated cortisol increases the risk for many health problems, including heart disease. Stress-induced cortisol secretion leads to not only stubborn belly fat but also a poorly functioning immune system and a lowered metabolism.

Surprising factors can lead to increases in your cortisol levels. For instance, how much cortisol do you think is contained in a cookie? While there isn't a measurable amount of the stress hormone itself hidden in that cookie, the sugar and refined flour that are there cause your body to stress out and secrete cortisol in response. How so?

Did you KNOW?

people who are **kind** have **23% less cortisol,** the stress hormone.

Imagine you are the driver of a finely tuned race car. The pit crew will make sure to add high-quality fuel for each race. However, if they put in regular gasoline, the kind you get at the local station, that car would be put under heavy stress due to the impurities, among other things, and start to break down. Much like adding poor-quality fuel to a race car, adding poor-quality food to your body causes your system to undergo stress.

Sleep deprivation has also been proven to increase cortisol levels. So if you are low on sleep, there is more happening than simply being irritated and constantly yawning. Losing a few Z's creates a domino effect because increased cortisol levels suppress your immune system. That explains why you're told to get rest when you're sick. It also explains why a long plane ride and trying to sleep in a new place can lead to a case of the sniffles.

Experts from the American Heart Association and the American Diabetes Association agree that excess belly fat causes fatty acids and hormones to be secreted into the liver, causing excessive amounts of glucose, which stresses your body out and elevates your insulin levels, leading to insulin resistance. This can lead right in to type 2 diabetes, leaving you vulnerable to other health conditions such as vision loss, heart disease, depression, nerve damage, gum disease, skin problems, circulation issues, and stroke. The fact is that diabetes can reduce your life expectancy, and it causes approximately 70,000 deaths annually in the U.S.

The good news is that, as your coach, I will show you the solution that will finally get rid of this dangerous, stubborn fat. In the next chapter, you will discover the reasons why **what you think can override nearly every other influencer of cortisol.** It comes down to the fact that a few simple yet powerful thoughts can dramatically reduce your stress, and thus the amount of cortisol produced.

You will effortlessly turn off your stress hormones, turn up your happiness, and curb your cravings, which subsequently increases your energy and allows your body to release up to 1.5 lbs. every day!

02

think fit™ and turn off stress

As I've already mentioned, stress can have cascading effects throughout the body. Experts have documented what high cortisol levels can lead to: You might not sleep well, so you'll be tired during the day. Your sex drive may suffer. Your immune system may also be kaput.

One of the biggest clues to your cortisol levels might be the size of your waist. Elevated levels of the stress hormone can make you crave unhealthy foods and gain weight—especially in your belly. Yet the way you look at the world and treat yourself can be a great indicator of how much stress you're feeling as well. In your life, is the glass half-full or half-empty? The way you answer that question could be another clue to your cortisol levels.

The Words We Say to Ourselves

To eliminate the most stubborn fat, reduce your stress and cortisol levels, and help you get your life back, let's discuss the first component of this program: Think Fit™.

Take a moment to think about the words you say to your children, your spouse, your parents, your friends. You undoubtedly tell them things like, "You can do it!" "You're fabulous!" and "I love you!" And I'll bet you're usually courteous, kind, and pleasant even to strangers in line at the grocery store.

Quick self-test: Have you honestly said these sorts of things to yourself recently? Probably not. And *that's* the secret saboteur that's been holding you back in your health goals! You

take the Stress Test

Generally, how are your sleeping habits?	(1) I do not sleep well. (2) I am sleeping okay. (3) I sleep very well.
How do you feel when you wake up?	(1) I am usually still tired. (2) I feel okay. (3) I wake up energized.
Are you experiencing weight gains or fluctuations?	(1) I am gaining weight, especially around my belly. (2) My weight is consistent, though higher than I'd like. (3) I am at, or steadily working toward, a healthy weight.
How often do you get sick?	(1) All the time! (2) I fall ill a few times a year. (3) I am rarely sick.
Do you experience food cravings?	(1) I often give in to cravings for junk foods. (2) My cravings for unhealthy foods are balanced. (3) I satisfy my body's cravings with healthy foods.
How often do you experience backaches and headaches?	(1) I often suffer from them. (2) I get an occasional headache or backache. (3) I rarely have a headache or backache.
How is your sex drive?	(1) It is very low or nonexistent. (2) It is okay, but could be better. (3) I am satisfied with my sex drive.
How often does your gut act up?	(1) My gut often troubles me. (2) I sometimes experience digestive upsets. (3) I have a healthy digestive system that doesn't act up.
How are your levels of anxiety?	(1) I often feel anxious. (2) I occasionally feel anxious. (3) I am content and rarely anxious.
How would you describe your general moods?	(1) I feel blue pretty often. (2) I am doing okay. (3) I generally feel happy.

**Each answer is worth the number of points to its left.
Tally up your points, and gauge your stress level on the following scale:**

26–30 points: You are doing pretty well and experience low levels of stress.
20–25 points: You are dealing with a moderate amount of stress.
10–19 points: You are suffering from a high buildup of stress.

may have been eating the right foods. You may have even been minimizing your vegging-out time on the couch. But you likely haven't given a thought to your thoughts.

Positive, supportive statements to yourself are known as *affirmations.* For my clients losing weight, I call my coaching messages and affirmations Think Fit™. They really do turn everything around on a biological level. It's hard to keep yourself in a negative, stressed mind-set when you're saying "I love you" or "You can do it!" Optimistic thoughts raise your levels of the hormone serotonin, which is a neurotransmitter that brings you feelings of calm and happiness. Levels in your body fluctuate due to age, sex, hormones, and many other factors.

Research from Carnegie Mellon University confirms that positive thoughts improve a person's ability to recover from stress. The results of one study showed that people under high pressure had impaired problem-solving skills; however, concentrating on a positive thought helped them break down the situation and focus on the issue at hand, thereby reducing stress.

In a 2009 study published in *Health Psychology,* the journal of the APA, researchers studied sympathetic nervous system responses to stress. They found that subjects who repeated self-affirmations were shielded from the effects of chronic stress. Researchers noted that the protective quality was actually strongest for those deemed the "most psychologically vulnerable." And Geoffrey L. Cohen at Stanford argues that affirming activities, such as repeating positive statements, remind people of "who they are" and trigger a defensive mechanism in the brain that renders stressful situations less threatening. All in all, when you change the words you say to yourself to be more positive, it can significantly reduce the amount of stress you are under and reduce side effects such as increased cortisol and belly fat.

Now, where I get really excited is hearing that positive thoughts have also been *proven to reduce carb cravings and bingeing,* which can be a big saboteur of many eating plans. This is why Think Fit™ is the missing key to making my plan work long-term, until it becomes a lifestyle. Increasing your serotonin levels with Think Fit™ helps with impulsivity, appetite, and food cravings. Carbohydrates help raise serotonin, so when your levels are low for whatever reason, your body looks for ways to fix that problem. It

Research shows that people who have regular support from an expert lose three times more weight than those who try to do it alone.

knows that eating sugar, carbs, and other unhealthy food is one of the easiest, though fleeting, ways to do so. That's why the cravings kick in.

However, a study done by researchers at the National Institute of Mental Health found that when people focus on future positive events, an area of their brain activates that *triggers serotonin production.* So instead of turning to carbs to raise your serotonin, you can simply make daily affirmations, or Think Fit™, part of your life. This will naturally increase your serotonin and reduce your carb cravings, while also decreasing your cortisol levels and feelings of stress!

Coaching and Support for Greater Results

Throughout this book, I discuss the importance of receiving support from your friends and family. Studies have found that social isolation leads to increased cortisol, while having more high-quality social connections reduces the stress hormone. I hope that you are able to find joy in your relationships, and your family and friends say kind words to you. In this book, I will also be providing daily support as your coach, and positively filling up your mind with empowering good thoughts through Think Fit™.

Coaching in particular is important for success: According to the Society for Public Health Education, people who have regular support from an expert lose three times more weight than those who got at it alone. One way that a coach can help guide you is by saying encouraging words that you can then internalize and repeat to yourself. A good coach would never say, "You did it wrong; you're worthless!" Of course not! Rather, he or she would say, "That was a good try, now let's adjust to make it better." The first statement is disheartening, while the latter is motivating and inspiring. After continuing to hear (or read) positive things from your coach, you can begin to say them to yourself.

Think about it: No one talks to you more than you "talk" to yourself. You can be your own best friend, or you can be your very worst enemy, depending upon the words you use with yourself. The thoughts that you think work directly on your subconscious. Getting coaching support through Think Fit™ will create a foundation in your mind for positive thoughts and lead to long-lasting results.

For example, the first week was a great breakthrough for my clients Jessica, Kelly, and Marian, and many others who wanted to lose more than 30 lbs.—they dropped anywhere from 4 to 12 lbs.! If you have similar weight-loss goals, these first seven days will be a huge step toward losing your stubborn belly fat. Clients of mine who wanted to lose less than 30 lbs. saw anywhere from 1 to 6 lbs. of fat lost in their first week. Your own results may vary from those of my clients, but I can guarantee a huge improvement in your mood and body composition within the first week.

Turn the page and get ready to discover the secret my clients have been using to be successful.

A Little Help to De-stress

Buried under massive amounts of stress and looking for a jump start? There are a few natural remedies that can help you stop stressing pronto. Gamma-aminobutyric acid (GABA) is an amazing neurotransmitter that helps you create a natural stress-free response. Another nutrient that you may be lacking is vitamin D. Though our bodies naturally source it from the sun, particularly during the summer months, vitamin D can also be supplemented to help your body regulate a stress-free day.

Omega-3s have been shown to keep stress hormones and levels of adrenaline under control. If you love fish, which is rich in this essential fatty acid, then it is easy to get the amount that you need; otherwise, supplements and enriched oils can be your "omega solution."

Another great stress fighter is vitamin C. Remember, however, that citrus fruits such as oranges are loaded with Sugar Calories, so reach for the lemons and limes or a vitamin supplement instead.

For more recommendations, including a list of supplements with my personal seal of approval, please turn to the Health Resources at the back of this book or visit JorgeCruise.com/Resources.

03

eat fit™ and lose 1.5 lbs. a day

Most of us understand that what we eat can control the numbers we see on the scale. With *Stubborn Fat Gone!*™, you will get my best recommendations on how to Eat Fit™ to lose your most difficult fat. However, before I share with you the foods lists and daily planners, you first need to know this: The dieting advice of the past 60 years has been WRONG, and it will be impossible for you to be successful by following the dieting advice of "Conventional Wisdom."

The common diet philosophy of calories-in versus calories-out has reigned supreme for decades, yet it continues to fail, and Americans continue to have issues with weight. Think for a second: If counting calories was the only thing that mattered, then you would be free to fulfill your daily requirements with six Snickers bars for 1,500 calories. However, compare the Snickers diet to that of somebody who eats more calories of salmon and spinach salads. Who would lose fat, who would be healthier, and who could sustain their diet? We don't need to count *all* calories, we really only need to count the calories that cause us to gain or lose weight—and that is from the foods that affect the hormone insulin.

Insulin is cortisol's partner in crime. It is the most important hormone that is responsible for helping your body know whether you should be burning fat as energy or storing it for later. Your body releases it into the bloodstream in response to sugar. Therefore, by paying attention to your sugar intake, you can avoid spikes of insulin and the signal to "store fat for the winter."

In my most recent books, I have outlined how specific foods are responsible for causing rises in this hormone. It is important to note that carbohydrates—even whole grains—can lead to insulin spikes. Harvard University states that "a starch is a long chain of sugar molecules." So, at a basic level, carbohydrates (even from so-called healthy sources) are just chains of sugar, which affect your insulin levels, causing you to gain weight and store fat. This is why I call the carbohydrates in foods **Sugar Calories.** These are the calories that truly affect weight gain, and the only ones you need to count.

With this program, I recommend eating no more than 100 Sugar Calories per day. This level is the best way to really maximize your health, helping you lose up to 1.5 lbs. each day and balance your hormone levels.

To calculate the number of Sugar Calories in an item, find the number of total carbohydrate grams on the nutrition label or look it up online. (Note that sugar grams are under the umbrella of total carbohydrates, so they don't need to be counted separately.) There are 4 calories per 1 gram of carbs, so to find the number of Sugar Calories, you just multiply the total grams of carbs by 4.

YOUR DAILY SUGAR CALORIE LIMIT IS:

100

Now, not everything that contains carbohydrates will count on this plan. The foods that I call **Freebies** either naturally have no Sugar Calories (for example, proteins such as chicken and fish) or they may have some carbohydrate grams but do not cause significant spikes in insulin, and therefore do not need to be counted (like broccoli). Maximize your Freebies to maximize your weight loss.

How to Eat

I have outlined exactly what you should eat for the next 12 weeks to help optimize your weight loss. You

what are
Freebies?

Freebies are the foods that do not cause significant spikes in insulin and therefore do not need to be counted toward your daily Sugar Calorie goal. They are healthy proteins, fats, and vegetables that are low in Sugar Calories and high in important nutrients.

Freebies actually work to help you get rid of belly fat rather than store it in your body.

the top 10
Freebies

1. Chicken
2. Eggs
3. Whipped cream
4. Greek yogurt
5. Broccoli
6. Almonds
7. Butter
8. Cheese
9. Half-and-half
10. Coffee, tea, water

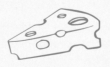

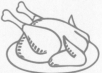

your inner Ecosystem

Believe it or not, your digestive system houses more than 500 different types of bacteria. While that may seem strange, your gut actually needs bacteria to keep your intestines healthy and help with digestion. Your inner ecosystem gets out of whack when the ratio of "good" to "bad" bacteria in your gut becomes unbalanced, leading to an excess of waste buildup, or what I like to call "false belly fat." It is important to eat probiotic-rich foods—such as yogurt and fermented vegetables like sauerkraut—to restore the good bacteria and flush out the false belly fat.

Taking a probiotic supplement is another great way to help restore your gut bacteria. My client Kerri, who was on *Steve Harvey* with me, had trouble with false belly fat when I first started working with her. She started taking probiotic supplements and was immediately restored. Visit JorgeCruise.com/Resources, or turn to the Health Resources section in the back of this book, for my probiotic recommendations.

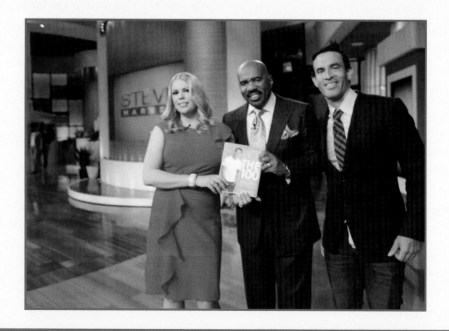

can find this in your daily trackers, which start in Chapter 6, where I tell you exactly what meal to eat each day and include the simple recipes you'll need. As I and many of my clients do, you will start each morning with a **Stubborn Fat Gone Shake** (recipe is at the end of this chapter), and then go on to have two balanced meals, two snacks, and a glass of red wine as a nightly treat.

I have also included Food Lists and a Bonus Recipe section so that you can branch out on your own if you'd like. However, I have done all of the work for you with my easy daily trackers, so I suggest following the menus as they have been laid out. You will notice that I've created 4 unique weeks of meals, which then repeat throughout the 12 weeks. I made sure to provide you with meals that you can easily toss together using common items you probably already have on hand. Simply follow my suggestions each day.

Note on the recipes: If there is no portion size listed for an ingredient, it is considered a Freebie and you can use as much or as little as you like. Make sure not to overeat and always stop if you are full, but there is no need to stress about portions if none are listed. And if a recipe says "season to taste," you may add as much as you like of

salt, pepper, herbs, or your favorite sugar-free spice. They are all Freebies.

The Food Lists

Foods that are lowest in Sugar Calories, especially the Freebies, help keep insulin levels low, leading to maximum weight loss. The following is a small guide to what foods are Freebies and what foods contain Sugar Calories. This is not an exhaustive list by any means, but it is a start.

The simplest thing to do is to follow each daily tracker, as all the work has been done for you. However, if you decide that you're going to count Sugar Calories yourself, check the Food Lists first. If there is something you can't find, remember that you simply need to multiply the number of total carbohydrate grams on any nutrition label by 4 (there are 4 calories for every 1 gram of carbohydrates) to get Sugar Calories.

If you're eating out, it is very common (and, in fact, the law in most places) for restaurants to provide nutrition information. If there is no breakdown of the total carbs for the meal, I suggest you order grilled chicken and grilled or steamed veggies.

These foods do not need to be counted toward your daily Sugar Calorie limit. They are *free*. These are foods that either naturally have no Sugar Calories (such as proteins) or do not cause significant spikes in insulin.

PROTEINS

Poultry

» Chicken breast
» Chicken deli meat
» Cornish hen
» Duck
» Goose
» Pheasant (no skin)
» Turkey bacon
» Turkey breast
» Turkey burger
» Turkey deli meat
» Turkey, lean ground

Eggs

» Chicken (brown or white)
» Duck
» Goose
» Whites (any kind)

Fish & Seafood

» Catfish
» Clams
» Cod
» Crab
» Flounder
» Halibut
» Lobster
» Mahi mahi
» Orange roughy
» Oysters
» Salmon
» Sardines
» Scallops
» Shrimp
» Sole
» Swordfish
» Tilapia
» Trout
» Tuna

Red Meat & Pork

» Bacon
» Beef (trimmed of fat), including:
  – chuck
  – cubed
  – flank
  – ground
  – jerky
  – porterhouse
  – rib
  – round, sirloin
  – rump roast
  – T-bone steak
  – tenderloin
» Bierwurst or beerwurst
» Bologna
» Buffalo
» Canadian bacon
» Capicola
» Chorizo
» Corned beef
» Deli & sandwich meats
» Devon (sausage)
» Ham
» Hot dog
» Lamb chop, leg, or roast
» Liverwurst
» Pastrami
» Pepperoni

- » Pork center loin chop
- » Pork roll
- » Pork tenderloin
- » Prosciutto
- » Roast beef
- » Roast pork
- » Salami
- » Sausage
- » Smoked meat
- » Summer sausage
- » Veal loin chop or roast

Other Protein Sources

- » Almonds
- » Almond butter, unsweetened
- » Almond flour/meal
- » Brazil nuts
- » Cashews
- » Jorge Cruise Protein Shake
- » Macadamia nuts
- » Pecans
- » Pine nuts
- » Pumpkin seeds

- » Stubborn Fat Gone Shake
- » Sunflower seeds
- » Tempeh
- » Tofu
- » Vegetarian hot dogs, such as Smart Dogs by Lightlife
- » Vegetarian meats, such as Chik'n by Morningstar Farms
- » Veggie burgers, such as Garden Veggie Patties by Morningstar Farms
- » Walnuts

VEGETABLES & FRUITS

- » Alfalfa spouts
- » Artichokes
- » Arugula
- » Asparagus
- » Avocado
- » Bell peppers: red, yellow, orange, or green
- » Bok choy, regular or baby
- » Broccoli
- » Brussels sprouts
- » Cabbage
- » Cauliflower
- » Celery
- » Collards

- » Cucumber
- » Eggplant
- » Endive
- » Fennel
- » Green beans
- » Green onion
- » Kale
- » Lemon
- » Lettuce, iceberg
- » Lettuce, red leaf
- » Lettuce, romaine
- » Lime
- » Mushrooms
- » Mustard greens

- » Okra
- » Onion
- » Pepper, jalapeño or serrano
- » Pickles, dill
- » Radicchio
- » Radishes
- » Scallions
- » Seaweed
- » Shallots
- » Snap peas
- » Spinach
- » Summer squash
- » Swiss chard

» Tomato
» Turnip greens
» Watercress
» Zucchini

HERBS & SPICES (FRESH OR DRIED)

» Basil
» Chives
» Cilantro
» Garlic

» Ginger
» Oregano
» Parsley
» Pepper

» Peppermint
» Salt
» Thyme

FATS

» Animal fats (lard, tallow, etc.)
» Avocado oil
» Butter

» Coconut oil
» Flaxseed oil
» Ghee

» Olive oil
» Sesame oil
» Walnut oil

DAIRY PRODUCTS

Cheese
» American
» Asiago
» Blue
» Brick
» Brie
» Cheddar
» Colby
» Colby Jack

» Cottage cheese
» Cream cheese
» Dry Jack
» Edam
» Farmer cheese
» Feta
» Fontina
» Gorgonzola
» Gouda

» Gruyère
» Havarti
» Limburger
» Mascarpone
» Monterey Jack
» Mozzarella
» Muenster
» Parmesan
» Pepato

» Pepper Jack

» Provolone

» Queso blanco

» Ricotta

» Romano

» Scamorza

» String cheese

» Swiss

» Teleme

» Greek yogurt (FAGE Total brand, recommended)

» Half-and-half

» Sour cream

» Whipped cream

MISCELLANEOUS

» Almond milk, unsweetened

» Baking powder

» Baking soda

» Blue cheese dressing

» Chia flour

» Coconut flakes and shreds, unsweetened

» Coconut flour

» Coconut milk, unsweetened

» Coffee

» Espresso

» Flaxseed, ground (Barlean's Forti-Flax, recommended)

» Flaxseed flour

» Flaxseed meal

» Hot sauce

» Italian dressing

» Mayonnaise

» Mustard

» Ranch dressing

» Salsa

» Sesame seeds

» Soy cheese

» Soy milk, unsweetened

» Soy sauce

» Sparkling water

» Stevia

» Stevita Tropical Singles (flavored stevia drink packs)

» Tea, unsweetened, hot or iced

» Truvia

» Vinegar: balsamic, white, wine

» Water

Here is a list of many common foods that are important to count. If a food you're looking for is not on the list, but is also not considered a Freebie, make sure to look up the total carbohydrate grams and multiply by 4 to get the Sugar Calorie total.

DAIRY PRODUCTS

Milk, 1% or fat free (1 cup) = 49 SUGAR CALORIES

Milk, nonfat dry (⅓ cup) = 12 SUGAR CALORIES

Milk, whole (1 cup) = 51 SUGAR CALORIES

Rice milk, plain, Rice Dream (1 cup) = 92 SUGAR CALORIES

Soy milk, plain, Silk (1 cup) = 32 SUGAR CALORIES

Yogurt, fat-free plain (6 oz.) = 52 SUGAR CALORIES

LEGUMES

Baked beans, original, Bush's Best (¼ cup) = 116 SUGAR CALORIES

Black beans, cooked (½ cup) = 92 SUGAR CALORIES

Chickpeas (garbanzo beans) (½ cup) = 65 SUGAR CALORIES

Edamame, shelled (soybeans) (½ cup) = 40 SUGAR CALORIES

Hummus (2 Tbsp.) = 16 SUGAR CALORIES

Kidney beans (¼ cup) = 40 SUGAR CALORIES

Lentils (¼ cup) = 40 SUGAR CALORIES

Pinto beans (¼ cup) = 44 SUGAR CALORIES

CARBOHYDRATES

Breads and Tortillas

Bagels, honey whole wheat (1) = 224 SUGAR CALORIES

Bread, sprouted whole grain (1 slice) = 60 SUGAR CALORIES

Bread, whole wheat (1 slice) = 88 SUGAR CALORIES

Hamburger bun (1) = 72 SUGAR CALORIES

Hamburger bun, sprouted whole grain (1) = 136 SUGAR CALORIES

Pancakes, frozen, ready-to-heat (4" diameter; 1) = 60 SUGAR CALORIES

Pita, whole wheat (1) = 62 SUGAR CALORIES

Roll, small dinner (1) = 52 SUGAR CALORIES

Tortilla, corn (6" diameter; 1) = 23 SUGAR CALORIES

Tortilla, flour (6" diameter; 1) = 64 SUGAR CALORIES

Waffles, frozen, ready-to-heat (4" diameter; 1) = 60 SUGAR CALORIES

Wrap, organic whole wheat (1) = 80 SUGAR CALORIES

Pasta

Penne, whole wheat, cooked (1 cup) = 208 SUGAR CALORIES

Spaghetti, whole wheat, cooked (1 cup) = 151 SUGAR CALORIES

Spirals, whole wheat, cooked (1 cup) = 149 SUGAR CALORIES

Cereals and Grains

Cereal, Cheerios (¾ cup) = 72 SUGAR CALORIES

Cereal, Ezekiel 4:9 sprouted whole grain (½ cup) = 160 SUGAR CALORIES

Cereal, Ezekiel 4:9 sprouted whole grain golden flax (½ cup) = 148 SUGAR CALORIES

Cereal, Post shredded wheat (1 cup) = 164 SUGAR CALORIES

Cereal, Total (¾ cup) = 92 SUGAR CALORIES

Cereal, Uncle Sam's (¾ cup) = 152 SUGAR CALORIES

Cereal, Wheaties (¾ cup) = 88 SUGAR CALORIES

Corn-muffin mix, "Jiffy" (¼ cup) = 108 SUGAR CALORIES

Couscous, cooked (½ cup) = 73 SUGAR CALORIES

Granola, low-fat (½ cup) = 160 SUGAR CALORIES

Oatmeal, dry steel-cut (¼ cup) = 108 SUGAR CALORIES

Oatmeal, Quaker instant apples and cinnamon (1 packet) = 88 SUGAR CALORIES

Oatmeal, Quaker original instant (1 packet) = 76 SUGAR CALORIES

Quinoa, cooked (½ cup) = 79 SUGAR CALORIES

Rice, basmati, cooked (½ cup) = 88 SUGAR CALORIES

Rice, brown, cooked (½ cup) = 92 SUGAR CALORIES

Rice, jasmine, cooked (½ cup) = 106 SUGAR CALORIES

Rice, Spanish, cooked (½ cup) = 80 SUGAR CALORIES

Rice, white, cooked (½ cup) = 106 SUGAR CALORIES

VEGETABLES

Acorn squash (½ cup) = 75 SUGAR CALORIES

Butternut squash (½ cup) = 43 SUGAR CALORIES

Corn, yellow or white (½ cup) = 58 SUGAR CALORIES

French fries, fast-food average (1 large) = 260 SUGAR CALORIES

Potato (1 medium) = 146 SUGAR CALORIES

Rutabaga, cubes (1 cup) = 58 SUGAR CALORIES

Sweet potato (1 medium) = 92 SUGAR CALORIES

Turnip, cubes (1 cup) = 34 SUGAR CALORIES

Vegetable blend, stir-fry frozen (¾ cup) = 20 SUGAR CALORIES

Yam (½ cup) = 75 SUGAR CALORIES

FRUITS

Fruits are healthy and have lots of vitamins—but they are primarily composed of Sugar Calories. I suggest choosing fruits with the fewest Sugar Calories, being mindful of portion sizes, and keeping servings to no more than two a day.

Apple (1 medium) = 99 SUGAR CALORIES

Apricot (1 medium) = 16 SUGAR CALORIES

Banana (1 medium) = 108 SUGAR CALORIES

Banana, dried (¼ cup) = 240 SUGAR CALORIES

Blackberries (½ cup) = 29 SUGAR CALORIES

Blueberries (½ cup) = 43 SUGAR CALORIES

Cantaloupe, cubed (½ cup) = 29 SUGAR CALORIES

Cherries (9) = 47 SUGAR CALORIES

Grapefruit, red or pink (½) = 21 SUGAR CALORIES

Honeydew (1 wedge) = 46 SUGAR CALORIES

Kiwi (1 medium) = 40 SUGAR CALORIES

Mango, sliced (½ cup) = 52 SUGAR CALORIES

Orange (1 small) = 45 SUGAR CALORIES

Peach (1 medium) = 59 SUGAR CALORIES

Pear (1 small) = 92 SUGAR CALORIES

Pineapple, diced (½ cup) = 43 SUGAR CALORIES

Plum (1 medium) = 30 SUGAR CALORIES

Raspberries (1 cup) = 59 SUGAR CALORIES

Tangerine (1 medium) = 47 SUGAR CALORIES

Tomato (1 medium) = 19 SUGAR CALORIES

Tomato, plum (1) = 10 SUGAR CALORIES

Tomatoes, cherry (½ cup) = 12 SUGAR CALORIES

Watermelon, diced (1 cup) = 46 SUGAR CALORIES

SNACKS & TREATS

Cheese puffs, Cheetos (1 oz.) = 60 SUGAR CALORIES

Chips, Doritos nacho cheese (1 oz.) = 68 SUGAR CALORIES

Chips, Kettle Chips, lightly salted (1 oz.) = 76 SUGAR CALORIES

Chips, Popchips, original (22 chips) = 80 SUGAR CALORIES

Chocolate, Green and Black's organic 85% dark (12 pieces) = 60 SUGAR CALORIES

Cookies, Joseph's, chocolate chip or oatmeal (4 cookies) = 52 SUGAR CALORIES

Cookies, Newman's Own chocolate crème (2 cookies) = 80 SUGAR CALORIES

Crackers, Nabisco Ritz, original (5) = 40 SUGAR CALORIES

Crackers, Nabisco Wheat Thins multigrain (6) = 88 SUGAR CALORIES

Crackers, Pepperidge Farms Goldfish (55 pieces) = 80 SUGAR CALORIES

Crackers, Wasa Original Crispbread (2 pieces) = 80 SUGAR CALORIES

Granola bar (1 bar) = 88 SUGAR CALORIES

Ice cream, soft serve, vanilla (½ cup) = 70 SUGAR CALORIES

Popcorn, air popped (3 cups) = 75 SUGAR CALORIES

Popcorn, kettle (1 cup) = 100 SUGAR CALORIES

Popcorn, Pirate's Booty (1 oz.) = 72 SUGAR CALORIES

Popcorn, Quaker rice cakes, lightly salted (2) = 56 SUGAR CALORIES

Trail mix (1 oz.) = 45 SUGAR CALORIES

BEVERAGES

Apple juice (8 oz.) = 116 SUGAR CALORIES

Beer, Coors Light (1 bottle) = 20 SUGAR CALORIES

Beer, Michelob Ultra (1 bottle) = 10 SUGAR CALORIES

Beer, Miller Lite (1 bottle) = 13 SUGAR CALORIES

Beer, O'Doul's, nonalcoholic (1 bottle) = 53 SUGAR CALORIES

Energy drink, Diet Rockstar (8 oz.) = 8 SUGAR CALORIES (but contains dangerous artificial sweeteners)

Energy drink, Red Bull, sugar free (8 oz.) = 11 SUGAR CALORIES (but contains dangerous artificial sweeteners)

Ginger ale, Schweppes (4 oz.) = 46 SUGAR CALORIES

Grapefruit juice, light, Ocean Spray (8 oz.) = 120 SUGAR CALORIES

Soda, Diet Coke (8 oz.) = 0 SUGAR CALORIES (but contains dangerous artificial sweeteners)

Soda, Steaz, organic sparkling green tea (1 can) = 92 SUGAR CALORIES

Sports drink, Gatorade, lemonade (4 oz.) = 30 SUGAR CALORIES

Vegetable juice, V8 100% (8 oz.) = 40 SUGAR CALORIES

Wine, dessert (1 glass, 5 oz.) = 80 SUGAR CALORIES

Wine, red (1 glass, 5 oz.) = 15 SUGAR CALORIES

Wine, white (1 glass, 5 oz.) = 15 SUGAR CALORIES

CONDIMENTS & DRESSINGS

Apple sauce, unsweetened (½ cup) = 56 SUGAR CALORIES

Barbecue sauce (2 Tbsp.) = 102 SUGAR CALORIES

Cocktail sauce (2 Tbsp.) = 30 SUGAR CALORIES

Honey (1 Tbsp.) = 69 SUGAR CALORIES

Ketchup (1 Tbsp.) = 15 SUGAR CALORIES

Miracle Whip, light (2 Tbsp.) = 24 SUGAR CALORIES

Peanut butter (2 Tbsp.) = 25 SUGAR CALORIES

Ranch dressing (2 Tbsp.) = 8 SUGAR CALORIES

Teriyaki sauce (2 Tbsp.) = 28 SUGAR CALORIES

Xylitol crystals (1 Tbsp.) = 24 SUGAR CALORIES

FROZEN FOODS

Amy's Frozen Meals

Black Bean and Vegetable Enchilada = 88 SUGAR CALORIES

Mexican Tofu Scramble = 160 SUGAR CALORIES

Shepherd's Pie = 108 SUGAR CALORIES

Spinach Feta Pocket Sandwich = 132 SUGAR CALORIES

Lean Cuisine Frozen Meals

Alfredo Pasta with Chicken & Broccoli = 148 SUGAR CALORIES

Baked Chicken = 120 SUGAR CALORIES

Beef and Broccoli = 172 SUGAR CALORIES

Beef Pot Roast = 100 SUGAR CALORIES

Chicken Marsala = 92 SUGAR CALORIES

Glazed Chicken = 104 SUGAR CALORIES

Grilled Chicken Caesar = 120 SUGAR CALORIES

Lemongrass Chicken = 152 SUGAR CALORIES

Meatloaf with Gravy & Whipped Potatoes = 100 SUGAR CALORIES

Roasted Chicken and Garden Vegetables = 140 SUGAR CALORIES

Roasted Chicken with Lemon Pepper Fettuccini = 112 SUGAR CALORIES

Roasted Garlic Chicken = 44 SUGAR CALORIES

Roasted Turkey & Vegetables = 72 SUGAR CALORIES

Rosemary Chicken = 116 SUGAR CALORIES

Salisbury Steak with Mac & Cheese = 92 SUGAR CALORIES

Salmon with Basil = 152 SUGAR CALORIES

Shrimp Alfredo = 116 SUGAR CALORIES

Shrimp and Angel Hair Pasta = 140 SUGAR CALORIES

Steak Tips Portobello = 56 SUGAR CALORIES

Stuffed Cabbage = 112 SUGAR CALORIES

Swedish Meatballs = 140 SUGAR CALORIES

Bonus Recipes

As I've said, I suggest sticking to the menus I laid out in your daily planner. If you do not like certain meals, feel free to experiment with the different foods on the Freebie Foods List. However, for a little variety, I've also included a few of my most popular recipes. Most serve more than 1, so they're great for sharing with your family or giving yourself plenty of leftovers!

ZESTY QUICHE LORRAINE

SERVES 4

15 Sugar Calories

6 eggs

¼ cup half-and-half

Tabasco Pepper Sauce or your
favorite hot sauce, to taste

¼ cup Swiss cheese, grated

3 green onions, green parts only,
thinly sliced

8 strips of bacon (or ½ cup ham
or pancetta, chopped)

Salt and pepper, to taste

Nonstick cooking spray

1 cup blackberries

Preheat oven to 350°F. Cook bacon, chop,
and set aside. Whisk the eggs, half-and-
half, and Tabasco until combined. Add the
cheese and green onions; season to taste
with salt and pepper.

Coat a 12-muffin tin with cooking spray.
Divide the bacon into each muffin cup and
top with the egg mixture. Bake for approximately 15–18 minutes or until a knife
inserted in the middle of the quiche comes
out clean. Let stand 5 minutes and serve.

Serve 3 quiches per person, with equal
amounts fruit on the side.

LOVELY LAYERED PARFAIT

SERVES 1

32 Sugar Calories

2 Tbsp. frozen raspberries,
unsweetened

1 Tbsp. Nature's Hollow Sugar-Free
Raspberry Preserves

2 Tbsp. frozen blackberries,
unsweetened

1 Tbsp. Nature's Hollow Sugar-Free
Wild Blueberry Preserves

½ cup FAGE Total Yogurt (Classic, 0%)

2 Tbsp. ground golden flax

Mix the raspberries with raspberry preserves in a bowl, and mix the blackberries with blueberry preserves in a
separate bowl. Build the parfait by lay-
ering in a glass: yogurt, blackberry mix,
yogurt, raspberry mix, yogurt. Top with
flax.

BLUEBERRY VELVET MUFFINS
SERVES 6

Freebie

Nonstick cooking spray

2 cups almond flour

2 tsp. baking powder

¼ tsp. salt

1/3 cup powdered xylitol

4 eggs

2/3 cup water

½ cup butter, melted

¼ cup Nature's Hollow Sugar-Free Wild
    Blueberry Preserves

SIDES:

6 Tbsp. Nature's Hollow Sugar-Free
    Wild Blueberry Preserves

6 pats butter

Preheat oven to 350°F. Coat a 12-muffin tin with cooking spray. Sift dry ingredients together in a large mixing bowl. In a small bowl, whisk together the eggs and water; stir in melted butter. Make a well in the center of the dry ingredients and pour in the wet ingredients. Mix until combined.

Fill the muffin cups ⅔ of the way full, and top each with 1 tsp. preserves; swirl preserves slightly with a toothpick. Bake for about 15 minutes or until a toothpick inserted in the center comes out clean.

Serve 2 muffins per person, with a pat of butter and a side of preserves.

ALMOND BREAD
MAKES 1 LOAF

Freebie

3½ cups almond flour

3 eggs

¼ cup butter, melted

1 tsp. baking soda

1 cup Greek yogurt (FAGE Total)

¼ tsp. salt

Preheat oven to 350° F. Mix together all ingredients in a bowl, then pour into a lightly greased bread pan. Bake for about 45 minutes. Remove from oven and let cool before removing from pan.

PECAN DELIGHT CHOPPED SALAD

SERVES 4

7 Sugar Calories

SALAD:

2 large chicken breasts, cooked
   and diced

1 bag (6 oz.) arugula, chopped

1 bag (6 oz.) baby spinach, chopped

½ cup raspberries

½ cup chopped pecans

½ cup Gorgonzola or goat cheese,
   crumbled

DRESSING:

½ cup extra-virgin olive oil

3 tsp. red-wine vinegar

1 packet stevia

1 tsp. Dijon mustard

1 tsp. chopped shallot

For the salad: Toss together the chopped arugula and spinach and divide evenly among 4 chilled salad bowls. Top with the remaining salad ingredients.

For the dressing: Whisk all listed ingredients until incorporated.

Serve each salad with a side of dressing.

FLAX FLAPJACKS

SERVES 1

Freebie

½ cup flaxseed flour

1 cup almond milk, unsweetened

4 egg whites

1 tsp. baking powder

2 Tbsp. almond butter

Butter or whipped cream, for garnish
   (optional)

Stir together all ingredients (except garnish) in a bowl until well combined. Pour desired amount into a greased, preheated skillet. Flip each pancake once.

Serve with butter or whipped cream, if desired.

LIGHTER SIDE CHEESY TURKEY BURGER

SERVES 4

Freebie

2 lbs. ground turkey

2 eggs, beaten

1 Tbsp. minced garlic

½ cup finely chopped onion

Salt and pepper to taste

8 slices cheddar cheese

2 Tbsp. mustard

2 Tbsp. Nature's Hollow
    Sugar-Free Ketchup

4 thin slices of tomato

4 thin slices of red onion

8 leaves green-leaf lettuce

Preheat grill to medium-high heat. Thoroughly combine the turkey, eggs, garlic, and onion. Divide meat and form into 8 patties; season with salt and pepper to taste. When the grill is ready, cook each burger about 4–6 minutes per side. Top each patty with a slice of cheese; close the grill and cook for 1 more minute or until the cheese starts to melt.

Stack two burger patties, spread with ketchup and mustard, then top with tomato and onion slices. Wrap between two leaves of lettuce and serve.

CRUNCHY SESAME CHICKEN SALAD

SERVES 4

16 Sugar Calories

SALAD:

3 cups romaine lettuce, shredded

2 cups Napa cabbage, shredded

½ cup red cabbage, shredded

2 large chicken breasts, cooked
   and sliced

1 cup sliced red bell pepper

1 cup soybean sprouts

½ cup Fresh Gourmet Authentic
   Wonton Strips

¼ cup slivered almonds

¼ cup thinly sliced green onion
   (optional)

1 Tbsp. black sesame seeds (optional)

DRESSING:

3 Tbsp. Eden Organic Brown Rice
   Vinegar

2 Tbsp. xylitol

2 tsp. soy sauce

1 Tbsp. sesame oil

¼ cup vegetable oil

Salt and pepper, to taste

For the salad: Toss the lettuce and cabbages together and divide evenly among 4 chilled salad plates. Arrange the remaining ingredients on the greens, reserving the green onions and sesame seeds (if desired).

For the dressing: Whisk all of the listed ingredients together, and season to taste.

Garnish each salad with green onions and sesame seeds, and serve with a side of dressing.

TANGY BBQ SALMON

SERVES 4

Freebie

FISH:

4 (6-oz.) wild-caught Atlantic salmon center-cut fillets

1 Tbsp. Old Bay Seasoning

½ cup Nature's Hollow Barbecue Sauce

Fresh dill sprigs, for garnish

SQUASH:

1 Tbsp. extra-virgin olive oil

2 garlic cloves, minced

2 cups sliced summer squash

2 cups sliced zucchini

½ cup white wine

For the salmon: Preheat grill to medium. Season the fillets with Old Bay and place on a hot, well-oiled grill. Cook for 4 minutes; turn and brush liberally with barbecue sauce. Cook for 5 minutes more; turn and brush with sauce, then turn once more and brush with sauce again. The fish is cooked when it flakes easily with a fork—do not overcook.

For the squash: Heat the oil and garlic in a medium skillet over medium heat. When the garlic is fragrant, add the squash and zucchini; sauté for about 7–8 minutes. Add the wine and simmer until the liquid has almost evaporated.

Serve the fish with the sautéed squash.

BOUNTIFUL STEAK FAJITA SALAD

SERVES 4

Freebie

FAJITA SALAD:

1 (16-oz.) rib eye steak

2 Tbsp. vegetable oil

½ cup sliced green bell pepper

½ cup sliced red bell pepper

½ cup julienned onion

1 fresh, sliced jalapeño

1 tsp. cumin

1 tsp. paprika

4 cups spinach

SIDES:

4 Tbsp. sour cream

4 Tbsp. La Victoria Salsa Suprema

4 Tbsp. Wholly Guacamole

Slice the rib eye into thin slices. Heat a large skillet over medium-high heat; add oil. When the oil is hot, add the steak and cook for 5 minutes, stirring occasionally. Add the peppers, onions, jalapeño, and seasonings; sauté until tender.

Divide the spinach evenly onto four plates. Serve the fajita mixture over a bed of spinach and top with 1 Tbsp. salsa, guacamole, and sour cream.

HOME-STYLE MEATLOAF

SERVES 4

5 Sugar Calories

MEATLOAF:

2 Tbsp. butter

½ cup grated carrots

½ cup chopped celery

½ cup diced onion

1 garlic clove, finely chopped

2 lbs. lean ground beef

2 large eggs

1 tsp. salt

1 tsp. pepper

1 tsp. dried oregano

2 Tbsp. Dijon mustard

½ cup Nature's Hollow Barbecue Sauce

BROCCOLI:

4 cups broccoli florets

¼ cup butter

For the meatloaf: Preheat oven to 350°F. In a saucepan, melt the butter over medium heat and add the carrots, celery, onion, and garlic. Sauté until onions are translucent and vegetables are soft; let cool. Once cooled, add the vegetables to a large bowl along with the next 6 ingredients; mix thoroughly by hand. Press into a well-oiled loaf pan and spread barbecue sauce over the top. Bake for 1 hour or until the internal temperature reaches 150°F. Remove and let rest for 10 minutes.

For the broccoli: Steam the florets for 6–7 minutes; toss with butter and season as desired.

Slice the meatloaf and serve, along with the steamed broccoli.

FRIED TOMATOES

SERVES 4 – 6

Freebie

2 tomatoes, sliced

2 eggs

2 cups coconut flour

Coconut oil

Salt and pepper, to taste

Heat coconut oil in a pan over medium heat. Beat eggs in a bowl. On a plate, mix the coconut flour with salt and pepper, to taste. Dip tomato slices in egg, then coat with the flour. Fry tomatoes in coconut oil until they are golden brown.

JORGE'S FRIED CHICKEN

SERVES 4

Freebie

4 chicken breasts, thinly sliced

3 eggs

2 cups coconut flour

Salt and pepper, to taste

Coconut oil (for frying)

½ cup blue cheese dressing

4 cups mixed greens

12 cherry tomatoes, chopped

Olive oil

Balsamic vinegar

Heat coconut oil in a skillet over medium heat. Beat eggs in a bowl. On a plate, mix the coconut flour with salt and pepper, to taste. Dip each chicken breast in the egg, then in the flour. Once covered with flour, dip the chicken in the egg again, then coat once more with the flour. Place chicken in hot oil and fry on each side until cooked thoroughly and golden brown.

Toss mixed greens and tomatoes with the olive oil and balsamic vinegar. Plate each chicken breast with an equal portion of salad and 2 Tbsp. of blue cheese for dipping.

JORGE'S CHOCOLATE LACE COOKIES

MAKES 12

Freebie

2 sticks butter, softened

2/3 cup Truvia Baking Blend

1 tsp. vanilla extract

2 large eggs

1 cup almond flour

¼ cup whey protein powder, unsweetened

¼ cup cocoa powder, unsweetened

1 tsp. baking powder

½ tsp. salt

4 oz. dark chocolate, chopped (86% cacao or higher)

1 cup walnuts, chopped

Preheat oven to 350° F. Line a baking sheet with parchment paper.

Mix together all ingredients in a large bowl, then spoon onto the lined baking sheet.

Freeze for 5 minutes, then bake 9–10 minutes.

Imagine a pro golfer getting ready to start his game, attempting to hit the ball while it's still in his bag. Of course you would think that this makes no sense. At the very least, he should take the ball out of the bag, and if he were smart he would place it on a golf tee. Being busy and starting your day without an easy, thought-out breakfast is like trying to hit a golf ball while it's still in the bag, and it can ruin your entire day.

When coaching my clients, I always emphasize a point that my mentor Dr. Oz shared with me: Automate a good breakfast!

Get ready to start your day energized and stress-free. New research has emerged from the University of Missouri, confirming that a high-protein breakfast will give your brain a significant boost. The study concluded that the protein gives you a greater feeling of satiation throughout the morning while keeping you more alert and activating neurotransmitters that make you feel good. Harvard has also chimed in, saying that increasing your protein intake will minimize your consumption of Sugar Calories throughout the day.

All this is wrapped up in one powerful shake that's a Freebie on my plan!

THE STUBBORN FAT GONE SHAKE

SERVES 1 | **Freebie**

1 scoop of shake mix

8 oz. Silk almond coconut milk blend, unsweetened

1 serving fiber blend supplement

Ice to desired thickness

OPTIONAL ADD-ONS:
Cold coffee
Raw cacao
Kale
Spinach
Almonds or almond butter
Cashews
Macadamia nuts
Flaxseeds
Chia seeds

Blend and enjoy!

Note: For the shake mix, follow package instructions regarding serving size. Use a blend that gives you 20g of protein per serving, which can be the Jorge Cruise Protein Shake or a mix of your choice. For shake mix and fiber supplement recommendations, flip to the Health Resources at the end of this book and visit JorgeCruise.com/Resources.

04

bonus: move fit™ to burn more stubborn fat

As a fitness trainer, my first recommendation is that you not incorporate exercise into your first week on this program. I've seen too many people who are just starting out make this mistake: they buy every supplement, purchase a gym membership, get the videos . . . and then on day 3 they are trying to take it all back. The best way to stick to a new program is through little steps. Get comfortable with Eat Fit™ and Think Fit™ first. Once you are on a solid routine, come back to this chapter to really maximize your results.

Good, now that you're back, I want you to forget what every trainer has told you about exercising specifically to target belly fat. You'll learn why the old equation of calories-in versus calories-out—creating a deficit in calories to lose weight—simply doesn't take enough into account.

Often when we think of a workout, we often envision a gym or personal trainers or running mindlessly on the road. While all of these have their place, what I am about to share with you is scientifically the fastest way to burn off belly fat. Exercising in short bursts of activity—known as high-intensity interval training (HIIT), or high-intensity intermittent exercise—actually allows you to *exercise less* while burning *more fat* than regular workouts! In a groundbreaking study published in the *International Journal of Obesity,* researchers found that women who did 20-minute sessions of HIIT three times a week lost more subcutaneous fat and improved their insulin resistance more than the group who exercised at a continuous, moderate pace for twice as long.

Dr. Stephen Boutcher, an esteemed expert on obesity and one of the researchers in the study, says that "numerous scientific studies do not support spot fat reduction." In other words, exercise causes fat from all over the body to be reduced, not just the areas you want to target. He points to elite tennis players to demonstrate this concept. If spot-reduction exercise were effective, he says, a player's racket arm should contain much less fat. However, researchers have shown that the while the racket arms of tennis players usually possess greater muscle and bone mass, both arms have similar levels of fat.

Numerous studies by Dr. Boutcher prove that HIIT is "more effective at reducing subcutaneous and abdominal body fat than other types of exercise." The visceral fat that surrounds your organs is also

"High-intensity intermittent exercise results in greater fat loss directly in the abdomen."

—Dr. Stephen Boutcher

known as "killer fat" because it is directly linked to poor health outcomes. Visceral fat has greater blood flow, so it is even more responsive to belly-fat loss than subcutaneous fat, which is located just under the skin.

How to Exercise

So here's what your HIIT routine will look like: you'll be alternating between 2 moves for 20 minutes, 3 days a week. After a 3-minute warm-up of your choice, you'll do a high-intensity move for 8 seconds, then an active-recovery move for 12 seconds, repeating for a full 20 minutes with no break. Follow this with a three-minute cool down, and that's it—you're done! Your body will be burning fat for hours and hours to come.

Your 8-second intervals are high-intensity, full-body moves that are designed to get your heart pumping. These are explosive movements that you'll be able to sustain for only a short time before moving on to the 12-second active-recovery exercise.

In active recovery, you'll be focusing on strength and endurance as opposed to cardio. Your heart rate should drop a bit so you can catch your breath, but you should still be working hard rather than resting. It will be tough, but this is your chance to spur your body to open up the fat-burning floodgates!

Over the next few pages, you'll find 6 options for your 8- and 12-second intervals that you can combine to create a simple, at-home routine. For even more variety in a fun, engaging, high-energy environment, please visit JorgeCruise.com.

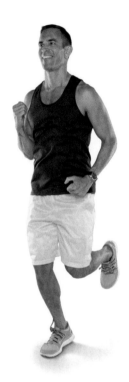 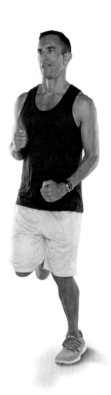

Start jogging in place, and go as fast as you can. To increase intensity, you can bring each knee up as you run—your thighs can go as high as being parallel to the ground. Engage your arms by moving them back and forth; this is an effective way to boost your heart rate even more.

12-Second Interval: Squats

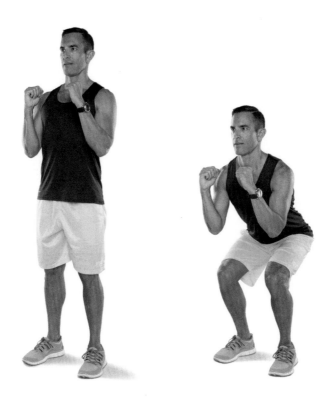

Keep your feet shoulder-width apart and place your arms up in front of you, shoulder height and parallel to the floor. Sit back, lowering yourself until your hips are at or below your knees. Pause for a second, then stand back up to starting position. Repeat for 12 seconds.

8-Second Interval: Lateral Shuffle

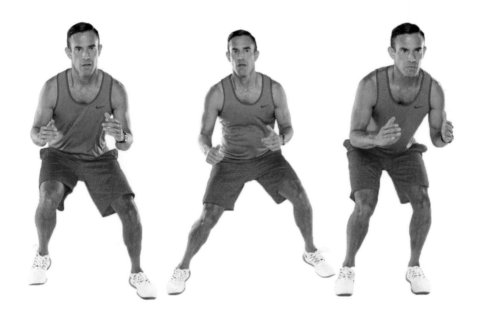

Begin with your hips square, and shuffle 4 steps sideways to the right. Keep your weight on your toes, moving as if there were a ladder to your side and you needed to step with both feet in each square. As you do so, mimic a running motion with your arms, moving your elbows back and forth. Try to keep your head straight and facing forward; avoid looking down as much as possible and try not to bend to either side. After taking 4 steps to the right, switch directions and shuffle to the left for 4 steps. Continue shuffling back and forth for the full 8 seconds.

12-Second Interval: Wide Squat

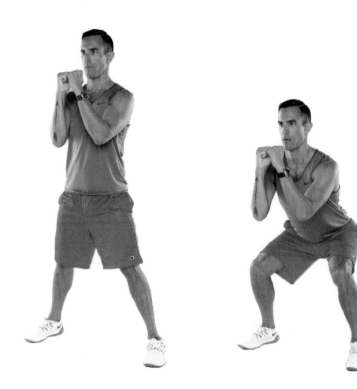

Stand with your feet slightly wider than shoulder width, with toes slightly pointed out. Have your hands in fists at chin height, elbows bent. Sit down, pushing your buttocks back and keeping your chest up, until your thighs are parallel to the floor. Pause for a second, then stand up quickly. Repeat for 12 seconds, trying to get lower with each squat.

8-Second Interval: Invisible Jump Rope

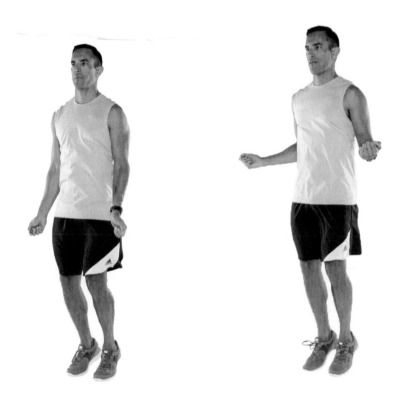

Stand up straight with a slight bend in your knees, hands by your sides. Quickly jump up and down on your toes and make small circular movements with your hands, as if you were using a real jump rope.

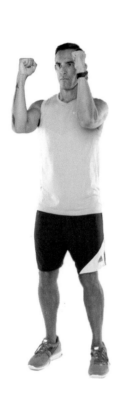
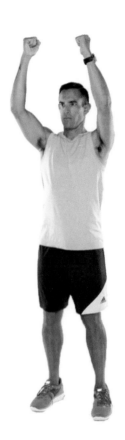

Stand with your feet shoulder-width apart. Make fists in front of your face, elbows at a 90-degree angle. Raise your arms up above your head, then lower your arms back to 90 degrees. Repeat for 12 seconds.

4 additional ways TO DO HIIT

The following are suggestions for taking your HIIT routine to the gym or outside. After an explanation of each workout and ways to adjust the intensity, there is a short sample workout. I've also included the intensity level you should be aiming for at each step on a scale from 1 to 10, with 1 being very little exertion and 10 being full exertion. To personalize the workout, adjust the incline, resistance, speed, etc., until your rate of exertion feels like it's at the right level for you. It might take a couple of tries to figure out the best high-intensity and active-recovery rates for you, but listen to your body and keep working.

Swimming

Swimming is not only fun, it may be the best way for those who suffer from knee or hip issues to hit those high levels of fat-burning intensity without experiencing any pain. What's also fantastic is that it can be done in a backyard pool almost as easily as in an Olympic or lap pool. While you won't have as much room to keep the "sprints" going in a small pool, you'll still get an intense workout by going back and forth more often.

Sample Workout

3-Minute Warm-up: 3 minutes of swimming laps at a comfortable pace (3–4 exertion).

8-Second Move: Freestyle sprint swimming (8–10 exertion).

12-Second Move: Light swimming or active paddling/treading water (6 exertion).

Alternate 8- and 12-Second Moves for 20 minutes.

3-Minute Cool Down: Easy laps (2–3 exertion).

Running

When it comes to the intensity of a running workout, your two options are to increase your speed and/or resistance. If you're running outside, you could make it tougher by running on soft, grassy terrain—or sand, for even more difficulty—rather than on pavement. This change throws a balance component into the mix, and in doing so can help make your 8-second bursts more challenging.

Sample Workout

3-Minute Warm-up: 3.5 mph with no incline (3–4 exertion).

8-Second Move: 6 mph at 2 percent incline (8–10 exertion).

12-Second Move: 4 mph at 2 percent incline (6 exertion).

Alternate 8- and 12-Second Moves for 20 minutes.

3-Minute Cool Down: 3.5 mph with no incline (2–3 exertion).

Elliptical

An elliptical is a great machine for low-impact cardio. During your high-intensity intervals, try to keep your heart rate at about 80 percent of its maximum. Your active-recovery intervals should keep your heart rate at about 50 to 65 percent of its maximum. To accomplish this on an elliptical, you can adjust the machine's resistance level or your rotations per minute (RPM), the speed that you're pushing the pedals.

Sample Workout

3-Minute Warm-up: Resistance 3, 40–50 RPM (3–4 exertion).

8-Second Move: Resistance 6, 80–100 RPM (8–10 exertion).

12-Second Move: Resistance 4, 50–60 RPM (6 exertion).

Alternate 8- and 12-Second Moves for 20 minutes.

3-Minute Cool Down: Resistance 2, 30 RPM (2–3 exertion).

Cycling

Using an exercise bike for your workout is an excellent option. Even the study at the beginning of this chapter on high-intensity interval training involved sprinting sessions on stationary bikes. A cycling workout is easier on your knees and other joints than running and jumping, which is especially important if exercise is a new endeavor for you or if you're severely overweight or obese. While the idea of actually sprinting may be daunting—or even impossible—completing your sprints on a stationary bike will yield excellent results without the stress and impact of running. To adjust the intensity of the exercise, change the machine's resistance level or your rotations per minute (RPM).

Sample Workout

3-Minute Warm-up: Resistance 3, 40 RPM (3–4 exertion).

8-Second Move: Resistance 10, 100 RPM (8–10 exertion).

12-Second Move: Resistance 6, 70 RPM (6 exertion).

Alternate 8- and 12-Second Moves for 20 minutes.

3-Minute Cool Down: Resistance 1, 40 RPM (23 exertion).

THINK ABOUT IT | **JUST A LITTLE MORE THAN 1 hr.** **A WEEK** **CAN BURN 2 lbs.**

1 HOUR

05

your 12-week guide

In these next 12 weeks, I will act as your personal coach, changing your thought patterns so you will finally release your stubborn fat. Why 12 weeks? The idea that you can change a habit in just 21, 28, or even 30 days is a fallacy. Ever notice the media reports of how often celebrities enter and exit recovery facilities? The problem is, these programs are usually too short. Scientists from the University College London who followed subjects as each tried to turn a new activity into a regular habit discovered that it takes an average of 66 days to make it stick, depending on what kind of habit is being formed. I encourage you to practice this new way of thinking for 84 days to ensure your success and really transform your mind with Think Fit™.

There are 84 daily entries of my Think Fit™ coaching sessions, each with a lesson, an affirmation to lock in what you are learning, and a motivational quote to further inspire you. Each week's lesson follows a theme to help you stay focused. Furthermore, every entry contains a tracker with my food and exercise recommendations for each day.

As you go through this 12-week Think Fit™ portion of the book, remember that the daily trackers and meal planners really make this a complete program for losing up to 1.5 lbs. every day and getting your body to a point of great health. It is important to do the readings and follow the eating plan to get the maximum benefit from this program. By following Think Fit™ alone, you would still lower your cortisol levels, increase your serotonin, curb cravings, and lose weight. However, as a complete plan for health and fitness, I encourage you to use all of the tools provided.

Think Fit™

Each night, starting tonight, I want you to sit down and do the Think Fit™ readings with me. I find the majority of people, including myself, struggle with cravings at night, so that is when I encourage you to read the lessons and find your motivation to "conquer the night." This book is your road map for your most successful journey, so do your best to keep it close to you for the next 12 weeks.

I'd like you to take the time to really think about each lesson and read the quotes. Repeat the affirmation as many times as you need—consider writing it down or putting it in your phone so you can look at it whenever you need the motivation boost. If you happen to be in a time of weakness, read the Think Fit™ message again and stay close to the encouraging, positive words.

Have a journal handy so that you can write down your responses to the questions and keep track of your thoughts and goals. You can also use it to copy down the affirmations and quotes that speak to you most. I have used journals ever since I can remember, and I keep them all to this day. It not only helps me process my thoughts and remember things, but I can also go back anytime I want and reflect on what my feelings or my goals were at a particular point in my life. If this sounds like something you would benefit from, I encourage you to do the same.

Eat Fit™

Who doesn't enjoy a delicious meal! You'll find my recommendations for what to eat in your daily trackers, and I encourage you to follow the menus exactly as I have laid them out for you. If I list an item without a portion size, it is considered a Freebie and the amount you use is up to your own discretion. All of the recipes are included in the daily trackers except for the Stubborn Fat Gone Shake, which is at the very end of Chapter 3, after the Bonus Recipes.

To keep things simple, I suggest the same breakfast every morning. My good friend and mentor Dr. Oz gave me the wonderful tip to "automate breakfast" for success, and I stick to that every day. Sometimes, however, I like to make a special breakfast, so I've included a few recipes that I personally use and like in the Bonus Recipes section of Chapter 3.

There are a few other features that will help you automate this plan. Each week I repeat meals, typically listing just three different lunch and dinner options. This way, you don't need to buy too many different things at the grocery store, and you can even make everything at once to save on prep time. I also completely repeat the weeks' menus every four weeks.

If you want to modify a menu, simply switch out one toss-together meal for another or create your own using the Food Lists and Bonus Recipes in Chapter 3. Simply make sure that you stay under 100 Sugar Calories daily. Check off what you eat in your tracker or write it down in your journal. If you ate something different from what I suggested, make sure to take note of the item and the number of Sugar Calories. Having this record will help keep you accountable.

This is the same eating plan I put my most successful clients on, so do your best to follow the recommendations each day, and it will keep things automated and enjoyable.

Bonus: Move Fit™

Remember: You can wait to exercise until after the weight has already begun to drop off. Don't put too much pressure on yourself by trying to learn everything at once. That said, getting the right workout in is easy with my high-intensity interval training program. Choose three days a week to do your 20-minute HIIT workouts, which will get your body burning belly fat as fuel. (I've noted recommended days in the tracker, for ease of use.) You can spend the other four days of the week doing whatever you like. You can take it easy and relax on the couch (you will still be using belly fat as fuel!) or you can do something else that you enjoy. If hitting the gym or lifting weights is up your alley, by all means do that. If you enjoy swimming, going for walks, or playing sports, those are all fine activities, too. You can even fit in more HIIT routines. Whatever you choose to do on these days, make sure that you really *enjoy* what you are doing.

After the 12 Weeks

After you have completed the 12 weeks, you will have worked to banish the negative thoughts you've been telling yourself, lowered your cortisol, raised your serotonin levels to increase happiness and combat carb cravings, balanced your insulin levels, and lost that stubborn fat. These 12 weeks will have helped you set up new thought, eating, and exercise habits until they became second nature. This new way of life should be ingrained in you. If you need suggestions for how to continue with your new habits so that they become your permanent lifestyle, consider any of the following:

— First, you can repeat the book. Do all 84 days over again. Continue to do Think Fit™ and follow my eating and exercise recommendations as they are laid out. This is a foolproof way to continue the positive changes you have made.

— If you don't want to repeat the entire book, memorize a few of your favorite affirmations and quotes. Use them to get centered whenever you feel stressed or are off track. Continue to use the meals and recipes, and keep doing the Move Fit™ workouts.

— Third, you can come to my website for more encouraging affirmations, exercises, food lists, and meal planners—all thought out for you! Please visit JorgeCruise.com to find out more.

No matter what path you take after the 12 weeks, I highly recommend that you connect with me and others on the plan for extra support by visiting Facebook.com/JorgeCruise.

Let's Begin!

Now that you understand how this book works, you are ready to hit the ground running! This book is like having me right next to you supporting your success, telling you that **you can do it.** If you are ready to stress less, boost your energy, and lose that stubborn fat forever, then let's begin!

06

lose stubborn belly fat *this* week!

Are you ready to make a change? Are you excited to start your new life? I hope that you feel all of the energy and enthusiasm of someone ready to embark on a wonderful journey—an amazing adventure!

Yet you're not heading to a far-off land or even to the beach. Your journey is to an even more interesting and exotic locale—yourself. What are your dreams and goals? What promises do you want to make to yourself? What are your biggest challenges, and what tools do you need to amass to overcome them? What is your true purpose in life?

Don't have the answers right this second? Don't worry! That's what Week 1 is all about. I wouldn't be surprised if you haven't really thought much about those things lately. Today

we are all so busy *thinking* and *doing* that we sometimes forget about *feeling.* With this book and Think Fit™ you're going to put it all together. After this journey of self-discovery, your thoughts, actions, and feelings will all work together in concert to help you release that stubborn belly fat.

And guess what? It's all going to begin this week. If you follow my program for just 7 days, you will begin to lower cortisol levels, have more energy than you've had in a long time, and start to look fabulous in your clothes again. You'll feel confident, vibrant, and alive. The changes you see in the mirror will literally mirror the changes that you feel on the inside.

I'm so excited for you to get started!

> *"A journey of a thousand miles begins with a single step."* — Lao-tzu

I HAVE
ALREADY TAKEN
THE FIRST
STEP.

Breakfast:

Snack:

Lunch:

Snack:

Dinner:

Treat:

Exercise:

Think Fit™

The Stubborn Fat Gone Shake

¼ cup almonds

Spinach Chicken Salad: Combine 1 sliced cooked chicken breast, 1 minced celery stalk, ¼ cup chopped almonds, 2 Tbsp. sour cream, 2 Tbsp. mayonnaise, 2 tsp. lemon juice, 2 Tbsp. Italian seasoning, and salt and pepper to taste. Toss together with 1½ cups spinach.

one hard-boiled egg

Signature Steak: Sauté ½ cup chopped onion, 1 chopped bell pepper, and 1 Tbsp. thyme. Reduce heat to low, add 2 Tbsp. dry red wine, and simmer a few minutes. Plate mixture with 3 oz. grilled flank steak and top with 2 Tbsp. crumbled goat cheese.

one glass red wine (15 Sugar Calories)
Not recommended during your first week.

Yesterday, last week, last year is gone. Today is the beginning of your new life—a new you! It's time for you to think about what this day and this journey mean to you.

I encourage you to think about this fresh start you're embarking on. Think about what a big deal this is. You've decided to make a life change. That's huge! Give yourself a hug or a pat on the back for committing to this change. Mark this occasion by drawing a star on your calendar, posting on Facebook, or telling a friend what you've decided to do. Making this statement is key.

Yesterday, and all of the yesterdays before it, are over. Today feel free knowing that you leave behind the diets and weight-loss struggles that let you down in the past. Today you begin the best part of your life, with new invigorating strategies and support that move you forward, pulling you where you want to go. Today is the day you start to shed that stubborn fat—for good.

Take a few minutes now to mindfully think about what this journey means to you and write down in your journal why you want to make this change.

> " *If you set goals and go after them with all the determination you can muster, your gifts will take you places that will amaze you.* " — Les Brown

I HAVE WHAT IT TAKES TO ACHIEVE MY GREATEST DREAMS.

Breakfast:

Snack:

Lunch:

Snack:

Dinner:

Treat:

Exercise:

Think Fit™

The Stubborn Fat Gone Shake

one string cheese

Bunless Burger: Use lettuce to wrap 1 cooked hamburger patty with ¼ sliced avocado, 5 slices cucumber, and mustard to taste.

cucumber slices with feta cheese

Lemon Grilled Salmon: Grill 1 salmon fillet, seasoned with lemon juice, salt, and pepper to taste. Serve with ½ cup steamed broccoli, seasoned to taste.

one glass red wine (15 Sugar Calories)

Not recommended during your first week.

If you don't know where you're going, how can you possibly hope to get to a destination? I'm a big believer in getting clarity and setting real goals. Personally, I have many ambitions for my own health and family life, and for helping clients. My most valuable realizations come when I start with my end target and work backward. I make sure that I have a series of achievable short-term goals so that I can build upon my success to reach the very big dreams of my long-term goals.

I want you to think about your own goals now, making sure to be specific. Rather than saying "I want to lose weight," say, "I want to lose 10 pounds from my belly and 2 inches off my waist." Write down your current and goal weight, waist measurement, and pant size. Our bodies can change in unexpected ways, so you might lose inches more quickly than pounds, or you might find that a pair of pants long relegated to the back of your closet will fit you sooner than a particular dress. Just remember to keep an eye out for success—of any kind.

CURRENT WEIGHT _____   CURRENT WAIST _____   CURRENT PANT SIZE_____

GOAL WEIGHT _____   GOAL WAIST _____   GOAL PANT SIZE _____

Write down some of your goals in your journal. Think about all of the reasons that they are important to you.

TRACKER

Breakfast:

Snack:

Lunch:

Snack:

Dinner:

Treat:

Exercise:

Think Fit™

"*Your body hears everything your mind says.*" — Naomi Judd

I TAKE GOOD CARE OF MYSELF.

The Stubborn Fat Gone Shake

celery sticks with almond butter

Chicken Sauté: Sauté 1 sliced chicken breast with ¼ cup red bell peppers, ¼ cup chopped onion, and ½ cup broccoli. Salt and pepper to taste.

¼ cup mixed nuts

Mushroom Pork Chop: Sauté 1 pork chop and top with ½ cup sautéed mushrooms. Serve with a side of ½ cup steamed broccoli. Season all with salt and pepper to taste.

one glass red wine (15 Sugar Calories)

Not recommended during your first week.

We make many promises to other people—both spoken and silent. We vow to our spouses to be faithful, we promise the company we work at that we'll do our best. We swear to our parents we'll be responsible, and we assure our children that we'll always love them. But what have you promised to *yourself?* If you're like most people, probably not much.

I encourage you right now to make a vow to yourself that you're committed to making changes for good health. Focus on keeping this promise to yourself, just as I'm sure you do when you promise something to people you love.

A promise is tricky because it can provide both comfort and stress. On the one hand, it offers security that something is likely to happen. On the other hand, you can't really guarantee that a promise will be fulfilled.

Honor this oath to yourself as if it were a fundamental component of who you are, like your eye color or height. I encourage you to review your promise to yourself each week, continually renewing your commitment to this new way of life.

Take a few minutes to mindfully think about the promises you need to keep for yourself. Write them down as well, so you will always have a reminder.

"There are always new, grander challenges to confront, and a true winner will embrace each one." — Mia Hamm

CHALLENGES EXCITE AND MOTIVATE ME.

Breakfast:

Snack:

Lunch:

Snack:

Dinner:

Treat:

Exercise:

Think Fit™

The Stubborn Fat Gone Shake

one string cheese

Spinach Chicken Salad: Combine 1 sliced cooked chicken breast, 1 minced celery stalk, ¼ cup chopped almonds, 2 Tbsp. sour cream, 2 Tbsp. mayonnaise, 2 tsp. lemon juice, 2 Tbsp. Italian seasoning, and salt and pepper to taste. Toss together with 1½ cups spinach.

cucumber slices with feta cheese

Signature Steak: Sauté ½ cup chopped onion, 1 chopped bell pepper, and 1 Tbsp. thyme. Reduce heat to low, add 2 Tbsp. dry red wine, and simmer a few minutes. Plate mixture with 3 oz. grilled flank steak and top with 2 Tbsp. crumbled goat cheese.

one glass red wine (15 Sugar Calories)

Not recommended during your first week.

When it comes to weight loss, there can be many challenges. Consider the smell of fresh doughnuts wafting out of a bakery. Or the homemade cookies your co-worker brought in to share. Or your spouse's well-meaning suggestion of "Let's go out for a nice dinner!" How about that leftover mac 'n' cheese sitting so temptingly on your child's plate?

Because we all have different strengths and weaknesses, some challenges will be, well, more challenging to you in particular than others. You might be able to pass up a serving of birthday cake at a party with no problem, but then find it hard to resist a bowl of potato chips. And therein lies the secret to your success: You can better overcome your struggles if you understand and prepare for the ones that are most difficult for you.

Be honest with yourself about when you are weakest. If that mac 'n' cheese has been a trigger, be sure to put away leftovers quickly. If baked goods are your weak point, keep Freebie snacks in your bag, desk, pocket, or car for those emergency situations. The point is to know where you might stumble and prepare ahead of time so you set yourself up for success.

It is time to really dig deep and identify your weight-loss challenges. Take a few minutes to think about your biggest struggles.

TRACKER

"Obstacles are those frightful things you see when you take your eyes off your goal." — Henry Ford

I HAVE INNER RESOURCES THAT CAN HANDLE ANY OBSTACLE I ENCOUNTER.

Breakfast:

Snack:

Lunch:

Snack:

Dinner:

Treat:

Exercise:

Think Fit™

The Stubborn Fat Gone Shake

¼ cup almonds

Bunless Burger: Use lettuce to wrap 1 cooked hamburger patty with ¼ sliced avocado, 5 slices cucumber, and mustard to taste.

one hard-boiled egg

Lemon Grilled Salmon: Grill 1 salmon fillet, seasoned with lemon juice, salt, and pepper to taste. Serve with ½ cup steamed broccoli, seasoned to taste.

one glass red wine (15 Sugar Calories)

Not recommended during your first week.

Now you have a pretty good idea what your weight-loss challenges are. Because knowledge is power, you can prepare for those challenges and meet them head-on.

However, I consider *obstacles* to be different from *challenges*. I think of challenges as things you know about ahead of time, things that you can plan ahead for. Obstacles, on the other hand, are those pesky things that just pop up without warning. You can't prepare for them because you can't foresee them coming.

When the obstacle is something in your life's path, especially one affecting your health, you can trust that the strength you need is inside you. When obstacles pop up, view them as an opportunity to practice creative solutions that will result in growth. Have faith in yourself. Don't wallow in self-pity; it's an energy-draining emotion. Instead, tap into your inner strength and resolve.

Even though you can't know what the next obstacle will be or when it will come, you can learn from your past success. Take a moment to reflect upon times you've faced obstacles. They don't have to be related to weight loss—they can be in the fields of work or relationships or what have you. What resources did you draw upon to overcome them? How can you apply the lessons you learned to future ones?

Write down some of your clever solutions to obstacles you've overcome.

> *"Do the best you can, and be good to yourself so that you can above all be good to others."*
> — Jessi Lane Adams

I WILL
TAKE TIME TO BE
SILENT AND
SEE MY TRUE
PURPOSE
IN LIFE.

TRACKER

Breakfast:

Snack:

Lunch:

Snack:

Dinner:

Treat:

Exercise:

Think Fit™

The Stubborn Fat Gone Shake

one string cheese

Chicken Sauté: Sauté 1 sliced chicken breast with ¼ cup red bell peppers, ¼ cup chopped onion, and ½ cup broccoli. Salt and pepper to taste.

cucumber slices with feta cheese

Mushroom Pork Chop: Sauté 1 pork chop and top with ½ cup sautéed mushrooms. Serve with a side of ½ cup steamed broccoli. Season all with salt and pepper to taste.

one glass red wine (15 Sugar Calories)

Not recommended during your first week.

While your main purpose for undertaking the Stubborn Fat Gone™ program may be to lose weight, components of the coaching will benefit you in myriad ways.

Reflect on what losing weight will do for you. How will it open you to the true purpose of your life? Take a moment right now simply to be silent and tune in to the great wisdom deep in the universe that speaks to you. Stop thinking, just for a moment, and listen. There are answers inside of you that can set you free. Your life gives you the opportunity to do good, help others, and spread kindness and love.

As for myself, I finally understood what losing one's health could mean when my father was diagnosed with cancer in 1986. My entire family felt shock when he was given only one year left to live, and this incident spurred me to take control of my health. Fortunately, my father is still alive, but that moment helped reveal to me that the purpose of my life is to help others find energy and vitality in their lives as I did.

Take a few minutes to meditate on *your* purpose in life.

> *"You yourself, as much as anybody in the entire universe, deserve your love and affection."*
>
> —Attributed to Buddha

I ACCEPT AND LOVE MYSELF JUST AS I AM.

Breakfast:

Snack:

Lunch:

Snack:

Dinner:

Treat:

Exercise:

Think Fit™

The Stubborn Fat Gone Shake

¼ cup almonds

Spinach Chicken Salad: Combine 1 sliced cooked chicken breast, 1 minced celery stalk, ¼ cup chopped almonds, 2 Tbsp. sour cream, 2 Tbsp. mayonnaise, 2 tsp. lemon juice, 2 Tbsp. Italian seasoning, and salt and pepper to taste. Toss together with 1½ cups spinach.

one hard-boiled egg

Signature Steak: Sauté ½ cup chopped onion, 1 chopped bell pepper, and 1 Tbsp. thyme. Reduce heat to low, add 2 Tbsp. dry red wine, and simmer a few minutes. Plate mixture with 3 oz. grilled flank steak and top with 2 Tbsp. crumbled goat cheese.

one glass red wine (15 Sugar Calories)

Not recommended during your first week.

Pop quiz: Would you love your mom more if she weighed less? Would you be kinder to your best friend if her BMI were lower? Could you feel happier with your child if she wore smaller clothes? Of course not! Your love for them isn't in any way tied to their waist measurement, BMI, or size. But what about your love for *yourself?*

The trick to real happiness is to stop beating yourself up for what you are not, and accept who you are right now. This is also the key to your ability to make more positive changes in your life. You deserve to be happy, and you deserve to love yourself, whatever your shape and size.

What do you like about yourself? What are your outstanding qualities that make you special? What are some instances where maybe you surprised yourself by showing extra kindness or goodness?

Take a few minutes to explore what this means for you. Love yourself as a mother loves her newborn baby. Be as kind to yourself as you are to your best friend. Show yourself compassion, nurturing, and tender care. Embrace and forgive yourself. It's the first path to freedom.

Forget the negative words you used to say to yourself. Instead, think about the new positive words you're going to be telling yourself from now on.

07

reach your goals

Welcome to Week 2 of your journey! Last week, you did a lot of introspection. I bet that you feel better acquainted with your wise, wonderful self than you have in a very long time.

This week, you'll move from focusing on your present to peering into your future. If you didn't change a thing, what would your life look like? Now focus the lens: What would your *ideal* future look like? While you can't change the past, you can always change your future. And the best way to do that is by setting goals.

You are the captain of the journey you're on, and you chart your course.

Just as a ship's captain uses navigation equipment—or even the stars—to follow a path, you will use the goals that you set. This week, you'll create goals for yourself: short-term, long-term, and everything in between. You'll discover the resources that you need to logically and skillfully navigate from your first target to the next, and then to the next.

Through reaching goal after goal after goal, you will be striding confidently in the direction of your dreams. Believe in yourself, and accept the challenge to better your health, your weight, and your life.

> "The secret of getting ahead is getting started. The secret of getting started is breaking your complex overwhelming tasks into small manageable tasks, and then starting on the first one."
>
> — Attributed to Mark Twain

I DESERVE THE HELP I RECEIVE IN MY LIFE.

TRACKER

Breakfast:

Snack:

Lunch:

Snack:

Dinner:

Treat:

Exercise (optional):

Think Fit™

The Stubborn Fat Gone Shake

celery sticks with almond butter

Chopped Salad: Top 2 cups chopped romaine lettuce with 1 chopped hard-boiled egg, ¼ diced avocado, ¼ cup diced tomatoes, 1 thinly sliced green onion, and ½ cup diced turkey breast. Dress with olive oil and vinegar.

¼ cup mixed nuts

Grilled Tilapia: Grill 1 tilapia fillet, seasoned to taste with lemon juice, salt, and pepper. Serve with ½ cup sautéed zucchini.

one glass red wine (15 Sugar Calories)

Do a high-intensity interval training workout.

Diets don't work. In fact, they are an *epic* failure. Research shows that 95 percent of all dieters gain back the weight that they'd lost within three years. So that means only 5 percent are successful at keeping the weight off—1 out of 20!

Why do diets fail? Sometimes it's because we're simply too busy, and the plan requires too much change initially, which leads to a sense of overwhelm and the desire to give up. Sometimes it's too restrictive, and we can't resist temptation.

So if diets don't work, what does? First off, it takes the right plan: a holistic approach that can become a lifestyle, not a fad. (Eating only cabbage soup or consuming only liquids are not healthy plans . . .) Along with that, changing your mind-set is key to staying consistent. In some ways, having powerful, supportive thoughts is even more influential on your weight loss than any diet you could follow. This perspective worked for me, and it will work for you. Having coaches—me, your friends, and yourself—will help you lose weight and will keep you going. Being the only person who is aware of and encouraging your change is a guaranteed failure.

Take a few minutes to think about how support, including having me as your coach, has made a difference during the past week.

> *"Setting goals is the first step in turning the invisible into the visible."* — Tony Robbins

I **EASILY** ACHIEVE WHAT I **SET OUT** TO ACHIEVE.

Breakfast:

Snack:

Lunch:

Snack:

Dinner:

Treat:

Exercise (optional):

Think Fit™

The Stubborn Fat Gone Shake

2 slices deli meat

Asian Chicken Salad: For dressing, combine 2 Tbsp. mayonnaise, 1 tsp. soy sauce, and ¼ tsp. lemon juice. In a separate bowl, combine 2 cups mixed greens with ½ cup diced, cooked chicken breast; ¼ cup chopped celery; and 2 Tbsp. chopped water chestnuts. Salt and pepper to taste.

2 slices cheddar cheese

Grilled Kebab: Briefly soak a wooden skewer in water. Alternate three 1" cubes of top sirloin, 3 slices red bell pepper, and 3 slices mushroom onto skewer. Season with salt and pepper, then grill over medium heat, turning halfway through cooking.

one glass red wine (15 Sugar Calories)

Today is a rest day.

Anyone can set a goal, then get distracted, lose interest, and never reach it. Consider New Year's resolutions. That's a popular time to set goals, right? I'm sure you won't be surprised to read that the top New Year's resolution year in and year out is to lose weight. Yet researchers at the University of Scranton found that only 8 percent of people end up achieving their New Year's resolutions. The other 92 percent give up!

Why are goals often unattainable for so many? Many of us abandon our dreams because they seem too big or too unreachable, but that just isn't true. Typically what happens is that when we don't see results in the timeline we expect, we assume that what we're doing isn't working. That is why I am such a believer in setting little goals you can reach up front. Then you can track your progress, build yourself up, and achieve success right at the start.

Let's say your goal is to love more or to live with passion each and every day. (Those are my personal starting goals.) First dream really big by creating an ideal image of yourself in the future, and then think of one small step that you can take toward that goal, something that would let you see results immediately.

Write down three to five specific goals, and take a few minutes to reflect on how you can start putting them into action right now.

> *"There is no chance, no destiny, no fate I Can circumvent or hinder or control I The firm resolve of a determined soul."*
>
> — Ella Wheeler Wilcox

I COMMUNICATE MY NEEDS WITH CALM CONFIDENCE AND GRACE.

Breakfast:

Snack:

Lunch:

Snack:

Dinner:

Treat:

Exercise (optional):

Think Fit™

The Stubborn Fat Gone Shake

celery sticks with almond butter

Lemon Chicken with Roasted Veggies: Preheat oven to 400° F. Season 1 chicken breast with 1 Tbsp. lemon juice, ½ Tbsp. olive oil, and salt and pepper. Place in greased baking dish and cook for 40 to 45 minutes. Serve with a side of ¼ cup sautéed mushrooms and ½ cup sautéed broccoli, seasoned to taste.

¼ cup mixed nuts

Portobello Pizzas: Preheat oven to 450° F. Grill 2 portobello mushrooms on both sides. Scoop out black fins and fill each mushroom with 1 Tbsp. pesto, shredded mozzarella cheese, black olives, and chopped cooked bacon. Sprinkle with Parmesan cheese and place in oven for 5 minutes.

one glass red wine (15 Sugar Calories)

Do a high-intensity interval training workout.

As you've already learned, *any* type of change—be it positive or negative—is hard. When you make changes to your lifestyle, to your health, it may be stressful for you, but it's also stressful for the people around you. For example, your co-workers might be used to going out with you for a celebratory lunch every Friday. Or your spouse might enjoy your Sunday-morning brunch. Or your kids might look forward to going to their favorite fast-food chain for weeknight dinners. If you're changing those types of things, it's only natural that these folks are going to be disappointed.

While some people may be supportive, others will resist. They might even unintentionally sabotage your efforts. Your co-workers might press a little harder to go to their favorite lunch spot; your spouse might complain about missing your usual brunch; and your children might whine about eating a meal cooked at home instead of handed out a drive-through window.

The challenge is that it's impossible to avoid everyone who might sabotage your weight-loss efforts! And since you can't avoid 'em, you're going to have to find ways to work with 'em. You need to find the resolve within yourself to stand firm, and you need to respectfully convey your wishes to those around you.

Take a few minutes to think of a time when you communicated with calm confidence and grace.

> "*Friends...they cherish each other's hopes. They are kind to each other's dreams.*" — Henry David Thoreau

MY **SUPPORT** CIRCLE WILL **HELP ME** SUCCEED AT WEIGHT LOSS.

Breakfast:

Snack:

Lunch:

Snack:

Dinner:

Treat:

Exercise (optional):

Think Fit™

The Stubborn Fat Gone Shake

2 slices deli meat

Chopped Salad: Top 2 cups chopped romaine lettuce with 1 chopped hard-boiled egg, ¼ diced avocado, ¼ cup diced tomatoes, 1 thinly sliced green onion, and ½ cup diced turkey breast. Dress with olive oil and vinegar.

2 slices cheddar cheese

Grilled Tilapia: Grill 1 tilapia fillet, seasoned to taste with lemon juice, salt, and pepper. Serve with ½ cup sautéed zucchini.

one glass red wine (15 Sugar Calories)

Today is a rest day.

We have discussed the importance of coaching and support—who is in your inner circle? (I thank you for having me as the chief in your tribe of weight loss.) It makes sense that the more support you have, the greater your success will be.

It's important to establish a network of people to help you on your health journey. It will be even more vital to your success to have those you can count on to hold you accountable and keep you going when times get tough. For your circle, select companions who live or aspire to live a healthy lifestyle. Having such people on your team will ensure you have solid support from those on the same path as you.

This group can include family members, co-workers, and good friends—anyone with whom you feel comfortable communicating openly and honestly. People on your inner support team must be caring and nonjudgmental; they must be willing to listen to you and support you.

Think of the names of three people you'd like to invite to be on your inner support team. Write their names down, and then be sure to let those individuals know how they can help you.

TRACKER

Breakfast:

Snack:

Lunch:

Snack:

Dinner:

Treat:

Exercise (optional)**:**

Think Fit™

"*When the student is ready, the teacher will appear.*" — Buddhist proverb

I AM
READY
TO BE
HEALED.

The Stubborn Fat Gone Shake

celery sticks with almond butter

Asian Chicken Salad: For dressing, combine 2 Tbsp. mayonnaise, 1 tsp. soy sauce, and ¼ tsp. lemon juice. In a separate bowl, combine 2 cups mixed greens with ½ cup diced, cooked chicken breast; ¼ cup chopped celery; and 2 Tbsp. chopped water chestnuts. Salt and pepper to taste.

¼ cup mixed nuts

Grilled Kebab: Briefly soak a wooden skewer in water. Alternate three 1" cubes of top sirloin, 3 slices red bell pepper, and 3 slices mushroom onto skewer. Season with salt and pepper, then grill over medium heat, turning halfway through cooking.

one glass red wine (15 Sugar Calories)

Do a high-intensity interval training workout.

That Buddhist proverb is one of my favorites. And it's especially apt for the journey you're on, which is so supported by coaching.

Today I want you to think about the different coaches you have had in your life. You might have called them "teachers" or "mentors." Perhaps they were your parents or grandparents, athletic coaches, community leaders, or even bosses. For me, I am incredibly grateful to my mother, who was so influential in my life.

For "extra credit," send one or two of your coaches an e-mail—or, better yet, a handwritten note—expressing your gratitude. I guarantee that doing so will make your day, and it may very well make their *month!*

When you are ready to be healed, the right teachers and coaches will appear for you. And they will be ready to help you, to heal you, so you can take your journey to the next step.

Take a trip down memory lane: spend a few minutes thinking of the names of five of your most influential coaches.

> "*Love yourself first and everything else falls into line. You really have to love yourself to get anything done in this world.*"
>
> — Lucille Ball

I AM
STRONG.
I KNOW
I CAN
DO IT!

TRACKER

Breakfast:

Snack:

Lunch:

Snack:

Dinner:

Treat:

Exercise (optional):

Think Fit™

The Stubborn Fat Gone Shake

2 slices deli meat

Lemon Chicken with Roasted Veggies: Preheat oven to 400° F. Season 1 chicken breast with 1 Tbsp. lemon juice, ½ Tbsp. olive oil, and salt and pepper. Place in greased baking dish and cook for 40 to 45 minutes. Serve with a side of ¼ cup sautéed mushrooms and ½ cup sautéed broccoli, seasoned to taste.

2 slices cheddar cheese

Portobello Pizzas: Preheat oven to 450° F. Grill 2 portobello mushrooms on both sides. Scoop out black fins and fill each mushroom with 1 Tbsp. pesto, shredded mozzarella cheese, black olives, and chopped cooked bacon. Sprinkle with Parmesan cheese and place in oven for 5 minutes.

one glass red wine (15 Sugar Calories)

Today is a rest day.

Hopefully, you're taking steps to avoid saboteurs, and you've stopped undermining yourself as well. If you're no longer being negative, that's terrific! But I don't want you to rest there—you shouldn't be neutral either! Today I'd like to see you actively start *supporting* yourself.

I bet that you're great at supporting other people. You cheer your children on at their games and encourage them to do well in school. You praise your spouse for doing well at work and probably even for picking up around the house. You listen to your friends talk about their successes, and you celebrate their wins with them.

But are you supporting yourself? When you meet a goal, do you give yourself the same level of care that you'd give to your friend, spouse, or child? Think about how you react when someone you love meets a goal, or even is just working really hard toward it. Then think about how you can offer that same enthusiasm to yourself.

Please embrace well-chosen supportive words about who you are. I can say without a shadow of a doubt that you are amazing. Deep down, you know that those wonderful beliefs about yourself are *true.* I want you to make encouraging yourself a practice in your daily life.

Take a few minutes to think about how you can celebrate your successes, and of the most supportive words you can say to yourself.

TRACKER

Breakfast:

Snack:

Lunch:

Snack:

Dinner:

Treat:

Exercise (optional):

Think Fit™

"The distance is nothing; it's only the first step that is difficult."

— Marie Anne de Vichy-Chamrond

I STEADFASTLY MOVE IN THE DIRECTION OF MY DREAMS.

The Stubborn Fat Gone Shake

celery sticks with almond butter

Chopped Salad: Top 2 cups chopped romaine lettuce with 1 chopped hard-boiled egg, ¼ diced avocado, ¼ cup diced tomatoes, 1 thinly sliced green onion, and ½ cup diced turkey breast. Dress with olive oil and vinegar.

¼ cup mixed nuts

Grilled Tilapia: Grill 1 tilapia fillet, seasoned to taste with lemon juice, salt, and pepper. Serve with ½ cup sautéed zucchini.

one glass red wine (15 Sugar Calories)

Today is a rest day.

Can you believe that we've arrived at the end of Week 2? Fourteen days of reflection, change, and growth. You made it!

Today take some time to look back on these past two weeks. You have accomplished a great deal: You decided to make a change. You made a commitment to yourself, your body, and your health. You set goals, and then you refined them. You identified challenges, obstacles, and saboteurs in your life, and you strategized ways to deal with them. Then you identified supporters in your life, and came up with ways to embrace them. Perhaps most important, you learned how to not be your own worst saboteur, and instead you learned how to be your own best supporter. You have taken so many steps—big and small—toward your dreams.

I can only assume that along the way you've had some challenges—that is to be expected! Remember that. No matter what happened this week, you need to embrace this as a new day and a fresh start. You've got this! Today is a new day.

Take a few minutes to think about what you've learned. How have you changed?

08

rebrand your kitchen the "fat-loss station"

Simply by using Think Fit™, you are going to lower your cortisol levels and lose belly fat. Your thoughts are *that* powerful. You don't need a calculator to add up calories, nor do you need to buy specialty equipment to pump iron. This component of the Stubborn Fat Gone™ program is so revolutionary because it can stand alone to activate weight loss.

But of course with a little support from the other components of the program, you can accelerate your weight loss and achieve greater health. Start with small changes in your routine. Try some of those simple things that you've always been "meaning to do" all along.

This week, I want you to take some time to think about your relationship with food. This will inspire you to make some changes within everyone's favorite room in the house: the kitchen. As you're thinking about food, the fuel for your body, you'll also be thinking about the fuel for your soul—your *passion.* What really feeds you?

> "*If you always do what you've always done, you'll always get what you've always got.*"
>
> — Robert J. Kursar

I AM CHANGING THE WAY I THINK ABOUT FOOD.

Breakfast:

Snack:

Lunch:

Snack:

Dinner:

Treat:

Exercise (optional):

Think Fit™

The Stubborn Fat Gone Shake

¼ cup sunflower seeds

Tossed Italian Salad: Toss together ½ cup steamed, chopped cauliflower; ½ cup steamed, chopped broccoli; 2 Tbsp. chopped red bell pepper; 3 sliced chopped ham; 2 Tbsp. olive oil; and salt and pepper, to taste.

one hard-boiled egg

Cheesy Turkey Burger: Top 1 grilled turkey burger patty with 1 slice provolone, 2 slices tomato, and 1 Tbsp. mustard. Serve on ¼ cup bed of arugula.

one glass red wine (15 Sugar Calories)

Do a high-intensity interval training workout.

The quote I have chosen for this day is one of my favorites. Interestingly, it's often attributed to both Mark Twain and Henry Ford. However, no matter who said it first, it surely bears repeating.

If you've struggled with your weight, you probably think about food—a lot. You might spend a lot of time thinking about when you can eat, what you "should" be eating, what you can't have, and so on. And after every meal or snack, the cycle continues, going on and on.

This week, let's remember that part of the process of creating healthy habits is changing the way we think and approaching things from a new perspective. Let's try to implement methods in our lives that promote a new way of living.

What is food to you? Do you see it as just sustenance? Is it a source of pleasure? Do you use it as a reward? Or for love?

For so many of us, food is not only something we enjoy, but also something we offer to ourselves as a reward, and something we offer to others as a symbol of our love. Being mindful about how you perceive and use food is the first step in your journey toward a new, healthier relationship with it.

Write down some of your thoughts about food, and brainstorm ways that you can reframe them in a healthier way.

TRACKER

Breakfast:

Snack:

Lunch:

Snack:

Dinner:

Treat:

Exercise (optional):

Think Fit™

"We cannot solve our problems with the same thinking we used when we created them."

— Attributed to Albert Einstein

I EAT TO LIVE.
I DO NOT LIVE TO EAT.

The Stubborn Fat Gone Shake

12 raw macadamia nuts

Shrimp Caesar Salad: Toss together 5 medium cooked shrimp, 2 cups shredded romaine, 5 cherry tomatoes, and 2 Tbsp. Caesar dressing.

2 slices salami spread with cream cheese

Dijon Chicken: Pan-fry 1 chicken breast, seasoned to taste and topped with 1 Tbsp. Dijon mustard. Serve with ¼ cup sautéed zucchini, seasoned to taste.

one glass red wine (15 Sugar Calories)

Today is a rest day.

Perspective is everything. To solve a problem, sometimes all you need to do is look at it in a new way. Have you ever lain on a floor and gazed up at something rather than looking at it head-on? It completely changes the way it appears.

Reread the affirmation for today. How does it apply to you? Up to now, you might have "lived to eat" because culturally, food is about so much more than sustenance. When we get together with friends and family—whether for joyous occasions, sad occasions, or no occasion at all—we eat. We go out to eat as a reward, to treat ourselves at the end of a long day or week. And, of course, we must feed ourselves and loved ones several times a day. Is it any wonder we think about food so much and it is often front and center in our lives?

Today shift your thinking so that instead of living to eat, you eat to live. What this means is that food will no longer be your focus; it is not the center of your attention. Instead, you allow your health and your life to be the star, and relegate food to a supporting role.

Take a few minutes to think about the ways that you eat to live. How can you choose food to fuel your body?

"*Prayer is when you talk to God. Meditation is when you're listening. Playing the piano allows you to do both at the same time.*" — Kelsey Grammer

I AM
FREE
IN THIS
SPACE.

TRACKER

Breakfast:

Snack:

Lunch:

Snack:

Dinner:

Treat:

Exercise (optional):

Think Fit™

The Stubborn Fat Gone Shake

¼ cup sunflower seeds

Blue Chopped Salad: Toss together 2 cups shredded romaine, 4 slices chopped deli turkey, 1 chopped hard-boiled egg, 2 Tbsp. blue cheese crumbles, and 2 Tbsp. blue cheese dressing.

one hard-boiled egg

Grilled Flank Steak: Grill to desired doneness one 3-oz. flank steak, seasoned to taste. Serve with a side salad of 2 cups spinach, 5 sliced cherry tomatoes, 2 Tbsp. feta cheese, and a dressing of olive oil and vinegar.

one glass red wine (15 Sugar Calories)

Do a high-intensity interval training workout.

Many activities can become meditative experiences when you bring the right mind-set to them. For many, cooking in the kitchen is a spiritual experience. It allows you to take time away from other activities, and bring your focus solely to cutting, slicing, chopping, sautéing, or broiling. Truly enjoying this time can transform your evening.

Stand in your kitchen and take a good look around for a few minutes. Do you feel comfortable and free to create? Identify any areas or items that stress you out, any projects that you've been "meaning to do" for ages, and the places that need organization. Throw out the items you never use, or have double of. Take charge of your creative zone.

If you share this space with others, be sure to discuss the changes you want to do before you give the kitchen a makeover. After you transform this area, you'll be able to really focus and meditate on the nutritious meal you are about to prepare, and fully enjoy the process.

Brainstorm some ways to reinvent your cooking space that will allow you to feel free to create. Write down ideas or sketch in your journal. Then go do it!

> *"The doctor of the future will give no medication, but will instruct his patients in the care of the human frame, in diet, and in the cause and prevention of disease."* — Thomas Edison

WHAT MY
HEART
FEELS
FUELS ME.

TRACKER

Breakfast:

Snack:

Lunch:

Snack:

Dinner:

Treat:

Exercise (optional):

Think Fit™

The Stubborn Fat Gone Shake

12 raw macadamia nuts

Tossed Italian Salad: Toss together ½ cup steamed, chopped cauliflower; ½ cup steamed, chopped broccoli; 2 Tbsp. chopped red bell pepper; 3 sliced chopped ham; 2 Tbsp. olive oil; and salt and pepper, to taste.

2 slices salami spread with cream cheese

Cheesy Turkey Burger: Top 1 grilled turkey burger patty with 1 slice provolone, 2 slices tomato, and 1 Tbsp. mustard. Serve on ¼ cup bed of arugula.

one glass red wine (15 Sugar Calories)

Today is a rest day.

By now, I hope you've begun changing your perspective so that you think of food as fuel. That's a huge paradigm shift—way to go! You eat to live, you don't live to eat; eating is what you do to sustain your body.

Today let's talk about what else you need to fuel you. Food fuels your body, but what fuels your soul? For me, my passion is helping others lead healthier lives. The fact that *you* are reading this book fuels my soul. The knowledge that I am motivating, encouraging, and helping others gets me up in the morning, propels me through the day, and allows me to rest easy at night. I then wake up bursting with energy, elated that I get to do it again!

What your heart feels is what is really, truly important to you. So, what is it? Today take a few minutes to think about what fuels your heart. What makes you feel both energized and at peace at the same time while you are doing it? *That's* the fuel for your soul!

A crust eaten in peace is better than a banquet partaken in anxiety." — Aesop

I **ENJOY** FOOD, AND I **TAKE TIME** TO **SAVOR** IT.

TRACKER

Breakfast:

Snack:

Lunch:

Snack:

Dinner:

Treat:

Exercise (optional):

Think Fit™

The Stubborn Fat Gone Shake

¼ cup sunflower seeds

Shrimp Caesar Salad: Toss together 5 medium cooked shrimp, 2 cups shredded romaine, 5 cherry tomatoes, and 2 Tbsp. Caesar dressing.

one hard-boiled egg

Dijon Chicken: Pan-fry 1 chicken breast, seasoned to taste and topped with 1 Tbsp. Dijon mustard. Serve with ¼ cup sautéed zucchini, seasoned to taste.

one glass red wine (15 Sugar Calories)

Do a high-intensity interval training workout.

Do you love food? I know I sure do! How do you usually consume it? Do you ever "enjoy" a meal by blitzing through and powering it down?

Today, take your time and savor your food. Dwell on the flavors, the smells, and the textures. Listen to your surroundings. Slow down and enjoy the experience. A mindful meal will be much more pleasant and deliver more satiety than one thoughtlessly eaten at a desk or in front of the television.

What mom hasn't told her kids, "Chew your food"? Turns out, this advice is right. Researchers in Japan recently showed a link between chewing food and calories burned. Study participants were divided into two groups, and each group got a certain amount of calories. Then they were told to first eat their food as quickly as possible, then to chew their food as much as possible before swallowing. The researchers showed that eating slowly and chewing thoroughly resulted in more calories burned.

I urge you to stop rushing through your meals. Be present in the moment and enjoy them.

Take a few minutes now to think about how being mindful in your eating—as well as in other areas of your life—can bring you more joy.

"*A man too busy to take care of his health is like a mechanic too busy to take care of his tools.*" — Spanish Proverb

I AM BLESSED WITH MANY TALENTS.

Breakfast:

Snack:

Lunch:

Snack:

Dinner:

Treat:

Exercise (optional):

Think Fit™

The Stubborn Fat Gone Shake

12 raw macadamia nuts

Blue Chopped Salad: Toss together 2 cups shredded romaine, 4 slices chopped deli turkey, 1 chopped hard-boiled egg, 2 Tbsp. blue cheese crumbles, and 2 Tbsp. blue cheese dressing.

2 slices salami spread with cream cheese

Grilled Flank Steak: Grill to desired doneness one 3-oz. flank steak, seasoned to taste. Serve with a side salad of 2 cups spinach, 5 sliced cherry tomatoes, 2 Tbsp. feta cheese, and a dressing of olive oil and vinegar.

one glass red wine (15 Sugar Calories)

Today is a rest day.

What would you consider your best quality? Are you creative? Smart? Resourceful? Loving? Think about how you can put your talents to use in response to one of the biggest challenges we all face: too little time. We have to do as much as we can in the minutes that we have.

The true key to weight loss can't be found in the gym or at the end of your fork— it's in your mind. So use it right now to brainstorm ways to save time and add more healthy habits to your days.

For example, I know that I am creative, and I love to come up with new ideas to help others. Mason jars have got to be one of my favorite tricks for organization and meal prep! You can store measured-out ingredients for a recipe in a Mason jar, and toss it together when you need to use it. Of course, the jars are also great for storing leftovers and more.

My favorite Mason-jar recipe is the "salad in a jar." Simply put the dressing at the bottom, then layer your salad ingredients in the same jar. Put heavier items on the bottom, and make sure that any items you don't want getting soggy (such as lettuce) are layered toward the top. Store in the refrigerator, and when you are ready to eat it, just shake up the jar and enjoy! It's a wonderful grab-and-go meal or snack.

Brainstorm some creative solutions to your own time-management and meal-prep challenges—mine was the Salad in a Jar.

"The mother's heart is the child's schoolroom."

— Henry Ward Beecher

I AM FULL OF PURPOSE.

Breakfast:

Snack:

Lunch:

Snack:

Dinner:

Treat:

Exercise (optional)**:**

Think Fit™

The Stubborn Fat Gone Shake

¼ cup sunflower seeds

Tossed Italian Salad: Toss together ½ cup steamed, chopped cauliflower; ½ cup steamed, chopped broccoli; 2 Tbsp. chopped red bell pepper; 3 sliced chopped ham; 2 Tbsp. olive oil; and salt and pepper, to taste.

one hard-boiled egg

Cheesy Turkey Burger: Top 1 grilled turkey burger patty with 1 slice provolone, 2 slices tomato, and 1 Tbsp. mustard. Serve on ¼ cup bed of arugula.

one glass red wine (15 Sugar Calories)

Today is a rest day.

If you have children, I'm sure you want the absolute best for them. It's important to keep in mind that the best time to start instilling healthy habits in your kids is when they're young. Research shows that this improves their chances of continuing these behaviors as adults. You're already off to a great start by modeling healthy living for them on your own weight-loss journey!

Focus on exposing your children to different things. Growing, developing bodies thrive on a nutrient-rich diet, which includes eating a wide variety of foods, especially vegetables. Don't get discouraged, though, if they don't jump at the chance to eat broccoli and brussels sprouts. Kids' taste buds and sense of smell are more sensitive than adults', so they can sometimes react squeamishly to a flavor the first time they encounter it. Many experts recommend first offering raw vegetables instead of cooked, so the smell won't be as strong. They also say it can take a child 10 to 12 tries of something before they start to like it, so be patient!

I know you accept your mission to model positive behaviors to help your family, especially your children, be healthy and strong!

Take a few minutes to think about the favorite healthy foods of each member of your family, and how you can prepare them more often.

09

boost your confidence

I bet that you are a perceptive person. You notice when your child seems a little "off" because of worries about school, your neighbors paint their shutters a different color, or your best friend changes her hair. However, like many of us, you might be less able to spot the changes in yourself. You may look in the mirror and somehow, as if dark magic were involved, don't see the new, 10-pounds-lighter you. Instead, you still see the same old bags and sags—even if they're no longer there.

It's time to start boosting your confidence and to start loving and believing in yourself. This week, you'll learn why dwelling on your challenges, your weight, and your health issues is counterproductive. To be free, you need to release the struggle.

Take some time right now to smash that old "magic mirror" and see yourself with new eyes. By this week, you've likely released a substantial percentage of your target fat loss. You might notice that your skin looks firmer and brighter, and you're feeling more energetic.

Look at yourself in the mirror again. *You* are the fairest one of all!

TRACKER

"*You have to love yourself. That's the single most powerful thing. Out of that springs: How are you eating? How are you exercising? How are you resting?*" — Nia Peeples

I RADIATE CONFIDENCE.

Breakfast:

Snack:

Lunch:

Snack:

Dinner:

Treat:

Exercise (optional):

Think Fit™

The Stubborn Fat Gone Shake

¼ cup pecans

Bacon Caprese Stack: Alternate 3 slices fresh mozzarella, 3 slices tomato, 3 strips cooked bacon, and 3 basil leaves in a stack. Drizzle with 1 Tbsp. balsamic vinegar.

one string cheese

Seasoned Salmon Spinach Salad: Rub one 3-oz. salmon fillet with butter and season with fresh dill. Grill, then serve atop 2 cups spinach with olive-oil-and-vinegar dressing.

one glass red wine (15 Sugar Calories)

Do a high-intensity interval training workout.

Do you ever stare when you see people who look like they have it all together, wondering, *How can I be more like that?* If you break down what's so captivating about them, you'll notice that they all carry themselves with confidence. They might not be perfect, but they represent the best "self" that they can be.

A great way to boost your confidence is to simply act "as if." Act as if you were already at your ideal weight. Act as if you had a million bucks. Act as if you thought you were the most amazing person on the planet—because you *are*.

Write down five of your best traits, ones that you are truly proud of. Walk tall knowing that you are amazing, and you radiate confidence.

"Optimism is the faith that leads to achievement; nothing can be done without hope." — Helen Keller

I **CAN** DO IT. THE **ONLY** OPTION FOR ME IS **SUCCESS.**

Breakfast:

Snack:

Lunch:

Snack:

Dinner:

Treat:

Exercise (optional)**:**

Think Fit™

The Stubborn Fat Gone Shake

¼ cup Brazil nuts

Crunchy Chicken Wraps: Sauté 3 oz. chopped chicken breast, 2 stalks finely chopped celery, ½ cup chopped scallions, ½ cup chopped water chestnuts, 2 Tbsp. sliced almonds, 2 Tbsp. soy sauce, and crushed red pepper to taste. Evenly divide cooked mixture between 8 romaine lettuce leaves, about 2 to 3 Tbsp. per leaf. Serve with a side of ½ cup mushrooms and 4 asparagus stalks sautéed with soy sauce.

celery sticks spread with cream cheese

Zucchini Puffs: In a bowl, mix 3 Tbsp. mayonnaise, 3 Tbsp. Parmesan cheese, 1 Tbsp. basil, and chopped garlic and lemon juice to taste. Spread mixture evenly over 2 sliced zucchini in a baking dish. Broil in oven for 1 or 2 minutes, until top is browned. Serve with a side salad of 1 cup spinach and 1 sliced tomato, dressed with lemon juice.

one glass red wine (15 Sugar Calories)

Today is a rest day.

If you ever have a crisis in confidence, take a moment to think about the person quoted here: Helen Keller. She was born both deaf and blind, and labeled "unteachable." However, with the help of her teacher, Annie Sullivan, she earned her bachelor of arts degree—the first deaf and blind person to do so—and published 12 books and several articles.

When I realized that I have complete confidence in my success, it was a wonderful turning point in my life. Whatever I set my mind to, I know I can achieve. And guess what—you can, too!

Imagine what you would do if you took failure out of the equation. If you knew that you could not fail, the only possibility would be success. When you look at things that way, you cannot lose. If you set your focus on something, that will surely be the outcome. So rather than thinking about failure, focus on what you desire. Think about, visualize, and talk about your success with friends and family. Suddenly, the only option for you will be success!

Take a few minutes now to reflect on situations when you thought you would fail—but instead succeeded.

> "I love the man that can smile in trouble, that can gather strength from distress, and grow brave by reflection." — Thomas Paine

I VALUE AND HONOR ALL I HAVE ACHIEVED AND ACCOMPLISHED.

Breakfast:

Snack:

Lunch:

Snack:

Dinner:

Treat:

Exercise (optional):

Think Fit™

The Stubborn Fat Gone Shake

¼ cup pecans

Broccoli Cheese Soup: Bring 2 cups chicken broth to a simmer, add 3 cups chopped broccoli, and cook until tender. In a separate pan, gently heat 4 oz. cream cheese and ¾ cup cream on low, stirring often. Purée broccoli mixture in a blender, then blend in cream-cheese mixture. Makes 4 servings; garnish each bowl with shredded cheddar cheese.

one string cheese

Spicy Taco Salad: Sauté ¼ lb. ground beef with 1 tsp. chili powder, ½ tsp. onion powder, and 1 clove minced garlic. Add to a bowl of 2 cups chopped salad greens, 1 chopped tomato, ½ chopped bell pepper, ½ sliced avocado, 1 Tbsp. sour cream, and 2 Tbsp. chopped cilantro. Top with 2 lime wedges.

one glass red wine (15 Sugar Calories)

Do a high-intensity interval training workout.

It's incredible to think that you're at Day 24. You've come a long way!

Today I want you to value and honor all that you have accomplished. You might be thinking. *Wait! Didn't you say not to look back because I'm not going that way?* It's true that I don't want you to dwell on the past, ruminating on old mistakes, thinking about things that didn't go quite as you'd hoped. However, it is helpful to *reflect* on your past in a positive way.

Take a few minutes now to reflect on how far you've come. Sit in a comfortable chair in a quiet room, and visualize the past 24 days. Remember the new habits you've developed. Think of the negative traits you've removed from your life. See your life's movie in your mind's eye, and acknowledge every time you made a decision that supported your new healthy life. Give yourself a mental pat on the back. Each of those moments in time represents growth and change.

"It is the sweet, simple things of life which are the real ones after all."

— Laura Ingalls Wilder

I **LOVE** MYSELF WITHOUT **COMPARING** MYSELF TO OTHERS.

Breakfast:

Snack:

Lunch:

Snack:

Dinner:

Treat:

Exercise (optional):

Think Fit™

The Stubborn Fat Gone Shake

¼ cup Brazil nuts

Bacon Caprese Stack: Alternate 3 slices fresh mozzarella, 3 slices tomato, 3 strips cooked bacon, and 3 basil leaves in a stack. Drizzle with 1 Tbsp. balsamic vinegar.

celery sticks spread with cream cheese

Seasoned Salmon Spinach Salad: Rub one 3-oz. salmon fillet with butter and season with fresh dill. Grill, then serve atop 2 cups spinach with olive-oil-and-vinegar dressing.

one glass red wine (15 Sugar Calories)

Today is a rest day.

We live in such a competitive society, where it seems like others are constantly keeping score. Who has the bigger house? Fatter paycheck? Flashier car? Some places even hold "diaper derbies" where infants are encouraged to crawl as fast as they can to win a race. Does that seem as nutty to you as it does to me? And as our children get older, they're graded in school and scored on the playing field.

We're taught from such an early age to compete, compare, and contrast. Indeed, many of us are so busy "keeping up with the Joneses" that we lose sight of what's really important in life. I believe it's time to get off of the competitive treadmill. Why are we all running so fast to go nowhere?

Rather than competing with each other, let's work together. I hope that you have gathered a supportive circle of family and friends around you, and you're not comparing how you're doing with how you perceive others to be doing. It doesn't matter if your friend wears a smaller size, your mother has lost more weight, or your sister makes more money. All that matters is you and *your* weight-loss journey, the changes you are making to better *your* life.

Repeat today's affirmation to yourself, and meditate on all the ways that you are incomparable.

> "Dream and give yourself permission to envision a you that you choose to be." — Joy Page

I GIVE MYSELF PERMISSION TO BE HEALTHY AND HAPPY.

Breakfast:

Snack:

Lunch:

Snack:

Dinner:

Treat:

Exercise (optional):

Think Fit™

The Stubborn Fat Gone Shake

¼ cup pecans

Crunchy Chicken Wraps: Sauté 3 oz. chopped chicken breast, 2 stalks finely chopped celery, ½ cup chopped scallions, ½ cup chopped water chestnuts, 2 Tbsp. sliced almonds, 2 Tbsp. soy sauce, and crushed red pepper to taste. Evenly divide cooked mixture between 8 romaine lettuce leaves, about 2 to 3 Tbsp. per leaf. Serve with a side of ½ cup mushrooms and 4 asparagus stalks sautéed with soy sauce.

one string cheese

Zucchini Puffs: In a bowl, mix 3 Tbsp. mayonnaise, 3 Tbsp. Parmesan cheese, 1 Tbsp. basil, and chopped garlic and lemon juice to taste. Spread mixture evenly over 2 sliced zucchini in a baking dish. Broil in oven for 1 or 2 minutes, until top is browned. Serve with a side salad of 1 cup spinach and 1 sliced tomato, dressed with lemon juice.

one glass red wine (15 Sugar Calories)

Do a high-intensity interval training workout.

What do you think of when you hear the word *permission*? It's funny, but I always think of the slips that children bring home from school for their parents to sign so they can go on a field trip or take part in an activity. It's such a formal word: someone in authority allowing someone else to do something.

Permission is a powerful thing, and today I want you to harness that power for yourself. I want you to give yourself permission to be healthy and happy. Doing so gives *you* the power! With these thoughts, you will feel that you have the ability within yourself to change your health and your life.

Today I want you to think about submitting your very own permission slip to yourself. You can simply repeat today's affirmation, but for "extra credit," you can design a more elaborate document. Get creative and spell out the details, such as granting yourself the time and money you need to exercise and prepare foods that fuel your body. Or you might give yourself the time off from household chores for a day to take a walk in nature with your best friend.

> " *A strong, positive attitude will create more miracles than any wonder drug.* " — Patricia Neal

EVERY
CHANGE
IN MY LIFE
LIFTS ME TO
NEW LEVELS.

TRACKER

Breakfast:

Snack:

Lunch:

Snack:

Dinner:

Treat:
Exercise (optional):

Think Fit™

The Stubborn Fat Gone Shake

¼ cup Brazil nuts

Broccoli Cheese Soup: Bring 2 cups chicken broth to a simmer, add 3 cups chopped broccoli, and cook until tender. In a separate pan, gently heat 4 oz. cream cheese and ¾ cup cream on low, stirring often. Purée broccoli mixture in a blender, then blend in cream-cheese mixture. Makes 4 servings; garnish each bowl with shredded cheddar cheese.

celery sticks spread with cream cheese

Spicy Taco Salad: Sauté ¼ lb. ground beef with 1 tsp. chili powder, ½ tsp. onion powder, and 1 clove minced garlic. Add to a bowl of 2 cups chopped salad greens, 1 chopped tomato, ½ chopped bell pepper, ½ sliced avocado, 1 Tbsp. sour cream, and 2 Tbsp. chopped cilantro. Top with 2 lime wedges.

one glass red wine (15 Sugar Calories)

Today is a rest day.

Take some time today to really look at yourself in the mirror. That can be daunting, I know, but I think you'll be pleasantly surprised. I bet you'll see your skin starting to look firmer—in fact, you're glowing! Do your eyes look brighter, more awake? Ask the people in your support circle what they notice about you, too.

As lovely as you might look, the changes you see in the mirror are just the tip of the iceberg! Far greater and more significant are the changes inside of you that you can't see—the improvement to your health.

Scientists know that a smaller waist can dramatically increase your lifespan. In a groundbreaking study published in November 2008 in the *New England Journal of Medicine*, researchers tracked more than 350,000 Europeans for nine years and revealed that having a high waist circumference almost doubles the risk of premature death, even in people who are not overweight! In other words, having too much belly fat can cut your lifespan in half. As little as two inches extra on your waist increases your mortality risk. Think of these first weeks on the Stubborn Fat Gone™ program as a down payment on a better, longer life.

Take a few minutes now to reflect on all of the exciting changes you see, both outside and in.

> "*A woman is like a tea bag. You can't tell how strong she is until you put her in hot water.*"
> — Attributed to Eleanor Roosevelt

I RELEASE THE STRUGGLE.

Breakfast:

Snack:

Lunch:

Snack:

Dinner:

Treat:

Exercise (optional):

Think Fit™

The Stubborn Fat Gone Shake

¼ cup pecans

Bacon Caprese Stack: Alternate 3 slices fresh mozzarella, 3 slices tomato, 3 strips cooked bacon, and 3 basil leaves in a stack. Drizzle with 1 Tbsp. balsamic vinegar.

one string cheese

Seasoned Salmon Spinach Salad: Rub one 3-oz. salmon fillet with butter and season with fresh dill. Grill, then serve atop 2 cups spinach with olive-oil-and-vinegar dressing.

one glass red wine (15 Sugar Calories)

Today is a rest day.

Change can be hard, can't it? My wish for you is that this time could be smooth and easy—but I know that probably isn't true. I know that these past few weeks, you've struggled to make these changes, and perhaps even fought against the idea that you needed to make them. It's human nature.

All too often, change can feel like a struggle. Our minds and bodies resist it. We love the status quo! What's the solution to a struggle? Just let go! When you release the struggle, when you aren't pushing, the universe isn't pushing back. When you relax, the universe relaxes with you. You feel less stress.

Try it for yourself. Take a few minutes today to sit in a quiet room and relax. If you can, meditate. I like to meditate a few days a week, and I am always so much calmer and more focused afterward. Yes, challenges strengthen you, but I think the real growth comes after the struggle is over. It's when we relax that we are truly able to grow stronger—and happier.

10

know that weight gain is not your fault

I've said it before, and I'll say it again: stubborn fat is *not your fault.*

Doesn't that thought feel liberating? Your body is physically programmed to store fat. Think about it: If your ancestors, their ancestors, and their far-off ancestors hadn't been able to store fat so they could make it through the lean times, you simply wouldn't exist today!

You are also mentally and emotionally programmed to store fat. However, as we've discussed, your thoughts have incredible power. You can use Think Fit™ to change your mind, along with your body, your health, and your life.

This week, we'll go deeper into changing your psychological programming so you can naturally maintain a lean body. You'll discover how to be truly kind to your body. You'll understand why your history isn't your destiny. You'll be motivated to change your future when you see how dramatically it impacts the future of your family—and even the future of your dearest friends.

This week is about empowering yourself and regaining control as you end compulsive, stress-related eating once and for all. You'll achieve a new confidence and clarity that will stay with you the rest of your days—not just in the form of vibrant health and weight loss, but in all areas of your life.

"*Nothing can bring you peace but yourself.*"

— Ralph Waldo Emerson

I BREATHE OUT FEAR.
I BREATHE IN SERENITY AND WISDOM.

TRACKER

Breakfast:

Snack:

Lunch:

Snack:

Dinner:

Treat:

Exercise (optional):

Think Fit™

The Stubborn Fat Gone Shake

¼ cup almonds

Spinach Chicken Salad: Combine 1 sliced cooked chicken breast, 1 minced celery stalk, ¼ cup chopped almonds, 2 Tbsp. sour cream, 2 Tbsp. mayonnaise, 2 tsp. lemon juice, 2 Tbsp. Italian seasoning, and salt and pepper to taste. Toss together with 1½ cups spinach.

one hard-boiled egg

Signature Steak: Sauté ½ cup chopped onion, 1 chopped bell pepper, and 1 Tbsp. thyme. Reduce heat to low, add 2 Tbsp. dry red wine, and simmer a few minutes. Plate mixture with 3 oz. grilled flank steak and top with 2 Tbsp. crumbled goat cheese.

one glass red wine (15 Sugar Calories)

Do a high-intensity interval training workout.

Do you ever feel fearful, stressed, or anxious? Silly question, right? We all experience fear, stress, and anxiety, and many of us look for the solution at the bottom of a potato chip bag. But guess what—it's not there!

When you try to solve your problems with food, it doesn't work. And to make matters worse, you'll then end up with another problem: excess weight and poor health. Remember, fear and stress causes your body to release cortisol, and this hormone in turn causes your body to hold on to that stubborn belly fat.

Of course you have stress, worries, fears, anxieties . . . I do, too! Instead of trying to eat my way through a situation, I have found far better ways to cope. Personally, exercise has always helped me break through the fog and feel great during times of anxiety. Whenever I'm stressed, I go for a simple jog outside or do something physical that I really enjoy.

Brainstorm healthy ways that you can use to cope with your fear, stress, and anxiety. It can be especially effective to use more than one strategy at once. For example, you might listen to soothing music while reading a good book in a bubble bath. That's three times the stress-busting power!

> "*Take care of your body. It's the only place you have to live.*"
>
> — Jim Rohn

I AM KIND TO MY BODY.

TRACKER

Breakfast:

Snack:

Lunch:

Snack:

Dinner:

Treat:

Exercise (optional):

Think Fit™

The Stubborn Fat Gone Shake

one string cheese

Bunless Burger: Use lettuce to wrap 1 cooked hamburger patty with ¼ sliced avocado, 5 slices cucumber, and mustard to taste.

cucumber slices with feta cheese

Lemon Grilled Salmon: Grill 1 salmon fillet, seasoned with lemon juice, salt, and pepper to taste. Serve with ½ cup steamed broccoli, seasoned to taste.

one glass red wine (15 Sugar Calories)

Today is a rest day.

If you are trying to lose weight, then by definition you aren't completely happy with your body. Sadly, some people take that a step further and actively *dislike* their bodies. I hope that you don't feel that way. Please don't do that to yourself!

Be kind to yourself. Respect your body. Above all, give your body a break! Did you know that most women's weight naturally fluctuates between 5 and 10 pounds each month? That's right, it's normal to put on weight because of hormonal changes and water retention. If you keep that in mind, you won't feel so discouraged by the number on the scale.

Think about how you feel about your body today, then compare that with how you want to feel about it in the future. If you have negative thoughts about your body, come up with positive reasons to feel grateful for it. Some examples might be: Your body gets you where you want to go. You have the strength to hold your baby or play with your children. Your body allows you to feel the sun on your face and the wind through your hair.

> *"I like the dreams of the future better than the history of the past."*
> —Thomas Jefferson

MY HISTORY IS NOT MY DESTINY.

Breakfast:

Snack:

Lunch:

Snack:

Dinner:

Treat:

Exercise (optional):

Think Fit™

The Stubborn Fat Gone Shake

¼ cup almonds

Chicken Sauté: Sauté 1 sliced chicken breast with ¼ cup red bell peppers, ¼ cup chopped onion, and ½ cup broccoli. Salt and pepper to taste.

one hard-boiled egg

Mushroom Pork Chop: Sauté 1 pork chop and top with ½ cup sautéed mushrooms. Serve with a side of ½ cup steamed broccoli. Season all with salt and pepper, to taste.

one glass red wine (15 Sugar Calories)

Do a high-intensity interval training workout.

Sometimes the past is more comfortable to contemplate than the future, isn't it? You can know what happened yesterday, last week, last month. The future is yet to come, and that can be scary.

Sometimes we try to hold on to the past, and we resist making changes that will better our future. Today I want you to reflect on some things that went right for you in the past, things that made you happy. Yes, those are wonderful memories, but I want you to remember that while your history might affect your future, it doesn't determine it. You have the power to learn from your past to change your present and improve your future.

I like to think of it like a flowchart. While an event in my past can affect my present, it is my choice whether to let it impact my future. For example, a few years ago I went scuba diving, and I loved it! I made wonderful memories with my sons and discovered another enjoyable way to be active. When I think of that positive memory today, I can choose to let it impact my future by planning another scuba-diving trip soon.

Now you try it! Take a few minutes now to think about the things you want to change—don't accept the idea that your history determines your future! What are some events in your past that you can use as a springboard for a more positive, healthy future?

"It is easier to build strong children than to repair broken men." — Frederick Douglass

MY CHOICES
IMPACT
MY CHILDREN'S
FUTURE.

Breakfast:

Snack:

Lunch:

Snack:

Dinner:

Treat:

Exercise (optional):

Think Fit™

The Stubborn Fat Gone Shake

one string cheese

Spinach Chicken Salad: Combine 1 sliced cooked chicken breast, 1 minced celery stalk, ¼ cup chopped almonds, 2 Tbsp. sour cream, 2 Tbsp. mayonnaise, 2 tsp. lemon juice, 2 Tbsp. Italian seasoning, and salt and pepper to taste. Toss together with 1½ cups spinach.

cucumber slices with feta cheese

Signature Steak: Sauté ½ cup chopped onion, 1 chopped bell pepper, and 1 Tbsp. thyme. Reduce heat to low, add 2 Tbsp. dry red wine, and simmer a few minutes. Plate mixture with 3 oz. grilled flank steak and top with 2 Tbsp. crumbled goat cheese.

one glass red wine (15 Sugar Calories)

Today is a rest day.

When you prepare a nutritious meal at home, lovingly dole out proper portions for your family, and sit down to savor good food and conversation, your children are watching. On the other hand, when you career through your day, slide through a drive-through like a NASCAR driver making a pit stop, toss a sack to your kids in the backseat, and eat a cheeseburger and fries while driving to soccer practice, your children are watching that, too.

Many parents find it incredibly motivating to know that their positive choices can help their children live healthier, happier, longer lives. Children and teens who regularly eat dinners with their parents are more likely to have healthier diets and be more well-adjusted than those who eat on their own.

So be a good role model and strengthen your family bond. Make sure you find time to sit and enjoy meals together. Perhaps you can even cook together! Share funny stories or interesting topics around the dinner table.

Take some time for your family today.

"Don't walk behind me; I may not lead. Don't walk in front of me; I may not follow. Just walk beside me and be my friend." — Attributed to Albert Camus

I AM WORTHY OF LOVE, SERENITY, AND JOY.

Breakfast:

Snack:

Lunch:

Snack:

Dinner:

Treat:

Exercise (optional):

Think Fit™

The Stubborn Fat Gone Shake

¼ cup almonds

Bunless Burger: Use lettuce to wrap 1 cooked hamburger patty with ¼ sliced avocado, 5 slices cucumber, and mustard to taste.

one hard-boiled egg

Lemon Grilled Salmon: Grill 1 salmon fillet, seasoned with lemon juice, salt, and pepper to taste. Serve with ½ cup steamed broccoli, seasoned to taste.

one glass red wine (15 Sugar Calories)

Do a high-intensity interval training workout.

You deserve to be happy, and you deserve to have friendships and the joy they bring. Ideally, some of your greatest supporters in your weight-loss journey are also your closest companions. However, did you know that several studies have found that your risk for obesity increases when you have overweight friends? A 2007 study published in the *New England Journal of Medicine* found strong links between a person's weight and the weight of their friends. An obese friend increases your risk of obesity by 57 to 171 percent, depending on the closeness of your relationship. A recent study from Arizona State University revealed that the reason for this link is that we unconsciously change our habits to mirror those of our friends.

If your friends are overweight, it's not your fault, but it doesn't need to be your problem either. Of course you don't love a person any less because of his or her clothing size. However, you can't let others' behaviors influence you on your way to great health. Concentrate on your own health journey; perhaps it will encourage your friends to make more positive choices as well.

Branch out and make new friends in places where people are making healthy choices, such as a park, gym, or health-food store. Having people in your social network who pay attention to their health will be encouraging for both you and your other friends.

Take a few minutes today to think about the healthy habits you want to bring into your life and the impact that may have on your friends, too.

> " *Our lives are the sum total of the choices we have made.* "
>
> — Wayne W. Dyer

I CELEBRATE
THE POSITIVE
CHOICES
I MAKE
TODAY.

TRACKER

Breakfast:

Snack:

Lunch:

Snack:

Dinner:

Treat:

Exercise (optional):

Think Fit™

The Stubborn Fat Gone Shake

one string cheese

Chicken Sauté: Sauté 1 sliced chicken breast with ¼ cup red bell peppers, ¼ cup chopped onion, and ½ cup broccoli. Salt and pepper to taste.

cucumber slices with feta cheese

Mushroom Pork Chop: Sauté 1 pork chop and top with ½ cup sautéed mushrooms. Serve with a side of ½ cup steamed broccoli. Season all with salt and pepper, to taste.

one glass red wine (15 Sugar Calories)

Today is a rest day.

Every single day, you make dozens of choices about your meals and snacks. While each decision on its own might not feel like a big deal, they all add up in time.

It's easy to overlook a handful of chips here and a few innocent M&M's there, but if you want to stay on track toward your goals, remember that every bite counts. Several small handfuls of Sugar Calories add up to too much, and it's easy to over-look how much you're eating if you snack mindlessly. If you want a treat, put the food on a plate and savor it. Practicing mindfulness and good portion control will prevent you from accidentally consuming too many Sugar Calories.

Today I want you to brainstorm ways to say no to bad food choices. Think of some of your favorite healthy foods that you can make your go-to snacks, and give them a place of honor in your pantry. For example, I love guacamole and cucumber slices, roasted mixed nuts, and cheese. Write your ideas in your journal.

> *"Man cannot discover new oceans unless he has the courage to lose sight of the shore."* — André Gide

CHANGE
BEGINS WITH
ME.

Breakfast:

Snack:

Lunch:

Snack:

Dinner:

Treat:

Exercise (optional):

Think Fit™

The Stubborn Fat Gone Shake

¼ cup almonds

Spinach Chicken Salad: Combine 1 sliced cooked chicken breast, 1 minced celery stalk, ¼ cup chopped almonds, 2 Tbsp. sour cream, 2 Tbsp. mayonnaise, 2 tsp. lemon juice, 2 Tbsp. Italian seasoning, and salt and pepper to taste. Toss together with 1½ cups spinach.

one hard-boiled egg

Signature Steak: Sauté ½ cup chopped onion, 1 chopped bell pepper, and 1 Tbsp. thyme. Reduce heat to low, add 2 Tbsp. dry red wine, and simmer a few minutes. Plate mixture with 3 oz. grilled flank steak and top with 2 Tbsp. crumbled goat cheese.

one glass red wine (15 Sugar Calories)

Today is a rest day.

You have now taken control of your weight, your health, and your life. You are bucking years of your history to make a fresh start for you, your children, and your children's children. *You* are the change!

It's time to check in with yourself and seriously analyze how much you have changed. You are retraining your mind and body to eat healthy food, to make good choices, to be strong and determined, and to be gentle and loving to yourself. I am so proud of the positive choices you've been making.

It can be scary to make major changes in our lives, whether with our health or something else. Generally, I like to try new things and seek out adventures. But change can sometimes be scary, even for me. When I feel uncertain about a choice I'm making, I take time to visualize the success that it will bring. I picture in my mind how everything will go, and I imagine how it will feel. I also make sure to check in with my support circle. If they agree that a decision is a good idea, I feel empowered to make it!

Change is not always easy, but it can bring so many positive things into our lives. Don't be afraid to "lose sight of the shore," as it says in today's quote. Instead, think of all the amazing possibilities on the other side!

Think for a few minutes about how you feel about change. Do you embrace it or loathe it?

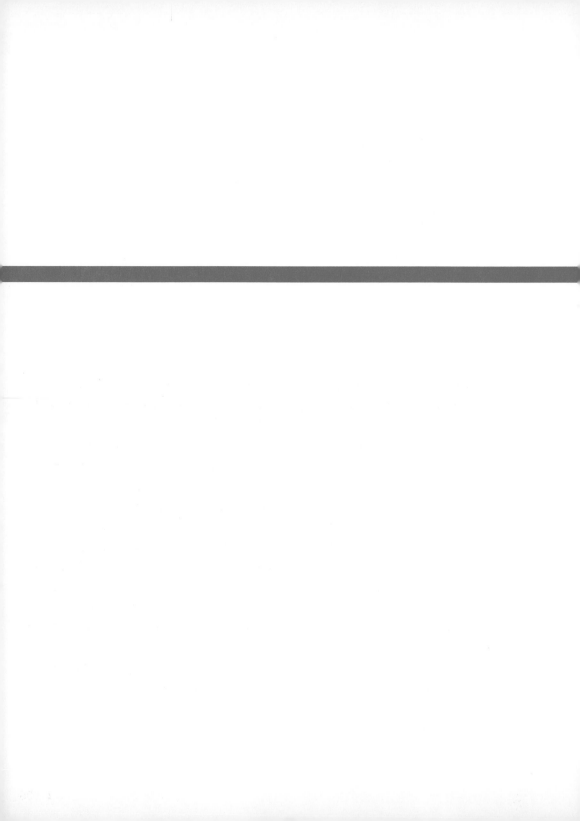

11

say *yes* to eating and going out!

Some things in life are universal. I feel confident that most people would agree that gathering with family and friends and going out to enjoy a delicious meal—one that you don't have to cook or clean up after—is a real treat!

You don't need to worry for a single nanosecond that you have to give up pleasures like eating out or taking vacations. Enjoying yourself isn't a luxury; it's a necessity!

I understand that the modern frenetic lifestyle requires fast food on the go, quick meals, and even frozen foods. But you can make positive, healthful choices about all of these things. This week, you will find the tools and the strength to do so!

We're also going to take some time to talk about something that I think is so critical to health and happiness. It's something you might not expect: appreciation. That's right, an "attitude of gratitude"—for your family and friends; for your community; and, and most important of all, yourself—is the key to your success. This week, we'll talk about how to tap into the spirit of appreciation and how to love and accept yourself.

Whether or not you have plans to go anywhere this week, we're about to embark on a journey of self-discovery. Ready? Let's go!

> " *Always do what you are afraid to do.* " — Ralph Waldo Emerson

I TAKE **POSITIVE ACTION** IN THE FACE OF **FEAR.**

Breakfast:

Snack:

Lunch:

Snack:

Dinner:

Treat:

Exercise (optional):

Think Fit™

The Stubborn Fat Gone Shake

celery sticks with almond butter

Chopped Salad: Top 2 cups chopped romaine lettuce with 1 chopped hard-boiled egg, ¼ diced avocado, ¼ cup diced tomatoes, 1 thinly sliced green onion, and ½ cup diced turkey breast. Dress with olive oil and vinegar.

¼ cup mixed nuts

Grilled Tilapia: Grill 1 tilapia fillet, seasoned to taste with lemon juice, salt, and pepper. Serve with ½ cup sautéed zucchini.

one glass red wine (15 Sugar Calories)

Do a high-intensity interval training workout.

Are there any temptations on your weight-loss journey that cause you fear? For example, some people dread being offered dessert at the end of a meal; others worry about facing the breadbasket or having to say no to a pastry with their coffee. At this point, can you face and conquer your fears? Assess your own strength and be sure not to overdo it. It is better to avoid putting yourself in a tempting situation in the first place rather than trying to tackle them too early and relapse.

When you're trying to make a selection at a restaurant, don't be afraid to ask for the nutritional info. Most restaurants are now required to provide it, and you can use this tool to make the best choices for your health.

Fear is not your friend. It increases your cortisol levels, causing you to hang on to that stubborn belly fat. You can release the fear—and the fat right along with it!

Take a few minutes to think about your favorite restaurants and look up nutritional information online to find a healthy go-to meal you can order at each one.

> "Two roads diverged in a wood, and I— / I took the one less traveled by, I And that has made all the difference."
>
> — Robert Frost

I TRUST MY INNER WISDOM TO MAKE HEALTHY CHOICES FOR MYSELF.

TRACKER

Breakfast:

Snack:

Lunch:

Snack:

Dinner:

Treat:

Exercise (optional):

Think Fit™

The Stubborn Fat Gone Shake

2 slices deli meat

Asian Chicken Salad: For dressing, combine 2 Tbsp. mayonnaise, 1 tsp. soy sauce, and ¼ tsp. lemon juice. In a separate bowl, combine 2 cups mixed greens with ½ cup diced, cooked chicken breast; ¼ cup chopped celery; and 2 Tbsp. chopped water chestnuts. Salt and pepper to taste.

2 slices cheddar cheese

Grilled Kebab: Briefly soak a wooden skewer in water. Alternate three 1" cubes of top sirloin, 3 slices red bell pepper, and 3 slices mushroom onto skewer. Season with salt and pepper, then grill over medium heat, turning halfway through cooking.

one glass red wine (15 Sugar Calories)

Today is a rest day.

Life is about choices, and some of the most difficult ones you'll be faced with on your weight-loss journey happen when you're away from all those healthy foods your kitchen is stocked with. It's hard to avoid restaurants and takeout forever. As our lives get busier and busier, the temptation to eat out or to order in gets stronger. In 1972, Americans spent $3 billion a year on fast food, while today we spend more than $110 billion. Eighty percent of Americans eat at a fast-food restaurant at least once a month.

When you order food, you'll be able to make better choices if you mentally prepare yourself first. Before you dive into the breadbasket or chips and salsa, pause and ponder whether it's really worth it. Think about how long you've been following your diet and how much weight you've lost. Remind yourself of the reasons you decided you needed to lose weight and get healthier. Research shows that taking time to think about your motivation will help you make healthier choices in the moment.

Today take a few minutes to think about your motivating factors for losing weight.

> "*The time to relax is when you don't have time for it.*"
>
> — Sydney J. Harris

I AM
REPAIRING,
REJUVENATING,
AND
REINVIGORATING
MY LIFE.

Breakfast:

Snack:

Lunch:

Snack:

Dinner:

Treat:

Exercise (optional):

Think Fit™

The Stubborn Fat Gone Shake

celery sticks with almond butter

Lemon Chicken with Roasted Veggies: Preheat oven to 400° F. Season 1 chicken breast with 1 Tbsp. lemon juice, ½ Tbsp. olive oil, and salt and pepper. Place in greased baking dish and cook for 40 to 45 minutes. Serve with a side of ¼ cup sautéed mushrooms and ½ cup sautéed broccoli, seasoned to taste.

¼ cup mixed nuts

Portobello Pizzas: Preheat oven to 450° F. Grill 2 portobello mushrooms on both sides. Scoop out black fins and fill each mushroom with 1 Tbsp. pesto, shredded mozzarella cheese, black olives, and chopped cooked bacon. Sprinkle with Parmesan cheese and place in oven for 5 minutes.

one glass red wine (15 Sugar Calories)

Do a high-intensity interval training workout.

We've talked a lot about change and the many positive choices you've been making. One way to look at it is that you're fixing and recharging your life; in other words, you're changing things for the better. Everyone's heard the expression, "If it ain't broke, don't fix it." I'd like to point out the flip side of that: "If it's broke, fix it!"

One way to repair, rejuvenate, and reinvigorate your life is to get away from it all and take a vacation. We certainly need it. Expedia.com conducts an annual "Vacation Deprivation" study and found that in 2013, Americans left an average of four vacation days unused, twice as many days as in the previous year. That adds up to an astounding 577,212,000 vacation days left un-enjoyed that year!

See if you can take a break and get away from it all for a week, a day, or even an hour. Whether or not you're able to take a vacation, try to add more laughter and levity to your life. Having fun and laughing actually reduces your cortisol levels, and many studies have proven the benefits to having a sense of humor.

Today I want you to think about how you are repairing, rejuvenating, and re-invigorating your life.

> "*Wherever you go, go with all your heart.*"
> — Confucius

I **KEEP** MY PROMISES TO MYSELF.

Breakfast:

Snack:

Lunch:

Snack:

Dinner:

Treat:

Exercise (optional):

Think Fit™

The Stubborn Fat Gone Shake

2 slices deli meat

Chopped Salad: Top 2 cups chopped romaine lettuce with 1 chopped hard-boiled egg, ¼ diced avocado, ¼ cup diced tomatoes, 1 thinly sliced green onion, and ½ cup diced turkey breast. Dress with olive oil and vinegar.

2 slices cheddar cheese

Grilled Tilapia: Grill 1 tilapia fillet, seasoned to taste with lemon juice, salt, and pepper. Serve with ½ cup sautéed zucchini.

one glass red wine (15 Sugar Calories)

Today is a rest day.

Many weeks ago, you made a promise to yourself. You promised to take good care of yourself and to make changes in your life to better your weight, your health, and your life. One of the biggest tests to your resolve comes with a break in your routine, such as when you go on a trip.

I love to travel, but it's one of the most challenging times for me to eat healthfully. The whole idea of a vacation suggests taking a break from life, and I'm surrounded by delicious, tempting foods.

So how do I deal with it? First, I always plan ahead. I Google restaurants in the area and try to take a peek at their menus. That way I can choose the healthiest options for me to eat at my leisure, when my willpower is strong because I'm not starving! As I decide on what to eat, I focus on the most healthful ingredients that I love, such as a crisp garden salad, fresh grilled salmon, and a flavorful cup of espresso.

You, too, can stick to your healthy habits. Today take a few minutes to brainstorm some ways to eat well when you're on vacation.

> *"No one realizes how beautiful it is to travel until he comes home and rests his head on his old, familiar pillow."* — Lin Yutang

I AM
AT HOME
WITH MYSELF
AND I AM
SAFE.

Breakfast:

Snack:

Lunch:

Snack:

Dinner:

Treat:

Exercise (optional):

Think Fit™

The Stubborn Fat Gone Shake

celery sticks with almond butter

Asian Chicken Salad: For dressing, combine 2 Tbsp. mayonnaise, 1 tsp. soy sauce, and ¼ tsp. lemon juice. In a separate bowl, combine 2 cups mixed greens with ½ cup diced, cooked chicken breast; ¼ cup chopped celery; and 2 Tbsp. chopped water chestnuts. Salt and pepper to taste.

¼ cup mixed nuts

Grilled Kebab: Briefly soak a wooden skewer in water. Alternate three 1" cubes of top sirloin, 3 slices red bell pepper, and 3 slices mushroom onto skewer. Season with salt and pepper, then grill over medium heat, turning halfway through cooking.

one glass red wine (15 Sugar Calories)

Do a high-intensity interval training workout.

Coming home can be a great opportunity to "reset" your life. Perhaps while you were away, you strayed a bit from your healthy habits. If you fell off the weight-loss wagon, it's time to climb right back on. Now that you're home, you can recommit to your promises to yourself. Get back to your usual schedule of eating well and exercising often. Try not to let too much time pass before you resume your normal activities.

Sometimes the best part of traveling is coming home. Breaking free from your routine might have made you appreciate your "regular" life all the more. You're back in familiar surroundings, surrounded by the things—and, more important, the people—you love.

More than just coming home, what does it mean to you to be at home with yourself? To me, it means that I feel comfortable with my own company. Take a few minutes today to reflect on what that means for you. Are you at home with yourself? If not, what can you do to change that situation?

> "The simple act of hopeful thinking can get you out of your fear zone and into your appreciation zone." — Martha Beck

EVERY DAY I APPRECIATE MYSELF MORE AND MORE.

Breakfast:

Snack:

Lunch:

Snack:

Dinner:

Treat:

Exercise (optional):

Think Fit™

The Stubborn Fat Gone Shake

2 slices deli meat

Lemon Chicken with Roasted Veggies: Preheat oven to 400° F. Season 1 chicken breast with 1 Tbsp. lemon juice, ½ Tbsp. olive oil, and salt and pepper. Place in greased baking dish and cook for 40 to 45 minutes. Serve with a side of ¼ cup sautéed mushrooms and ½ cup sautéed broccoli, seasoned to taste.

2 slices cheddar cheese

Portobello Pizzas: Preheat oven to 450° F. Grill 2 portobello mushrooms on both sides. Scoop out black fins and fill each mushroom with 1 Tbsp. pesto, shredded mozzarella cheese, black olives, and chopped cooked bacon. Sprinkle with Parmesan cheese and place in oven for 5 minutes.

one glass red wine (15 Sugar Calories)

Today is a rest day.

I hope that after yesterday's discussion you've gained a new appreciation for your life. Today I want you to gain a new appreciation for *yourself*.

What does it mean to appreciate yourself? It's not the same thing as loving yourself or respecting yourself. To appreciate yourself is to recognize your worth. I think the best way to do that is to take a few minutes to think of all that you are worth—all that you offer. First think about your various roles: Are you someone's child? A parent? A spouse? An employee or an employer? Now for each of those roles, consider what you offer. Do you comfort your children when they're sick? Help them with their homework? Do you offer help to your own parents in the form of financial support or love? Do you cook them nutritious meals for your spouse and family?

Continue to think about every one of the roles you play; I'm sure you're going to have a long list. If you write them down, you'll see the incredible number of things you offer in your life, and I guarantee that you'll feel tremendous admiration for yourself. As well you should!

> " *The greatest gift that you can give to others is the gift of unconditional love and acceptance.* "
>
> — Brian Tracy

I **APPROVE** OF MYSELF.

Breakfast:

Snack:

Lunch:

Snack:

Dinner:

Treat:

Exercise (optional):

Think Fit™

The Stubborn Fat Gone Shake

celery sticks with almond butter

Chopped Salad: Top 2 cups chopped romaine lettuce with 1 chopped hard-boiled egg, ¼ diced avocado, ¼ cup diced tomatoes, 1 thinly sliced green onion, and ½ cup diced turkey breast. Dress with olive oil and vinegar.

¼ cup mixed nuts

Grilled Tilapia: Grill 1 tilapia fillet, seasoned to taste with lemon juice, salt, and pepper. Serve with ½ cup sautéed zucchini.

one glass red wine (15 Sugar Calories)

Today is a rest day.

I hope that you've discovered a new appreciation for wise, wonderful you! Today we'll take that to the next level. Do you accept yourself? Another way to look at this question is: do you *approve* of yourself?

When I think of the word *approval,* it's hard not to think of *seal of approval.* There's a formality there. To really approve of yourself, I think you need to take a step back. What do you see when you assess yourself from a bit of a distance?

Some experts say that our own self-approval is the key to having a happy life. This makes complete sense to me. Once you accept yourself, then you can stop seeking approval from other people because you already know that you are enough. It's from that space of comfort and freedom that you will be able to stretch, challenge yourself, and strive to live your best life.

A round of applause for you! You have now completed six weeks on your weight-loss journey! What are the three biggest things you have gained or lost from this program so far?

12

keep stubborn fat off in a pinch!

By asking this, I'm probably dating myself, but do you remember those old cereal commercials that referred to the fat on your body by asking if you could "pinch an inch"? That phrase used to stick in my head, and even thinking about it now, it still makes me cringe! This week, we're going to banish all those negative thoughts like that about our bodies. Instead, we're going to replace them with positive thoughts with the power of Think Fit™.

It's so ironic that some of the most pleasurable things in life present some of the largest challenges to weight loss and good health. By now, I bet you've realized that it's relatively easy to eat well when you're in the comfort of your own kitchen and have complete control of what's in the cupboards and fridge. Similarly, you've probably found that it's easier to stick to Think Fit™ when you're home, where you feel loved and safe. You're able to keep positive messages at the forefront of your mind and integrate these ideas into your days.

But what about when you take the show on the road? You aren't the food shopper for the local zoo, nor do you stock the food court's pantry at the mall, nor do you plan the menu for a friend's party! You don't have much control over any of these situations.

Before you venture outside of your day-to-day to events like these, you need to restock your supplies of willpower. And this week, we'll brainstorm ways to do just that. You can do it; you can keep that stubborn fat gone!

"Everything negative—pressure, challenges—is all an opportunity for me to rise." — Kobe Bryant

I AM EQUIPPED TO HANDLE ANY NEW SITUATION—NO MATTER HOW DIFFICULT.

Breakfast:

Snack:

Lunch:

Snack:

Dinner:

Treat:

Exercise (optional):

Think Fit™

The Stubborn Fat Gone Shake

¼ cup sunflower seeds

Tossed Italian Salad: Toss together ½ cup steamed, chopped cauliflower; ½ cup steamed, chopped broccoli; 2 Tbsp. chopped red bell pepper; 3 sliced chopped ham; 2 Tbsp. olive oil; and salt and pepper, to taste.

one hard-boiled egg

Cheesy Turkey Burger: Top 1 grilled turkey burger patty with 1 slice provolone, 2 slices tomato, and 1 Tbsp. mustard. Serve on ¼ cup bed of arugula.

one glass red wine (15 Sugar Calories)

Do a high-intensity interval training workout.

I think that some of the most difficult challenges in life are the new ones. They're things you haven't encountered before, so you might not know how to react. That makes them especially challenging because you can't possibly know what you don't know! How can you prepare for the unexpected?

As an example, consider taking a trip with your family to a zoo, the county fair, or the beach. You've never been there, so you don't know what healthy food options there will be—if any. Here are my preparation strategies: If you're going somewhere that allows you to pack your own food, skip the vendors and do just that. Pack a backpack or small cooler with water, string cheese, almonds, boiled eggs, celery sticks, and perhaps even a small salad with grilled chicken. Portion out everything in baggies, and bring enough for the family. You'll save lots of money, and you'll lose weight to boot.

Take a few minutes to think about some of your favorite pack-along snacks.

"*You have power over your mind— not outside events. Realize this, and you will find strength.*" — Marcus Aurelius

I GROW
MORE INTUITIVE,
INSPIRED, AND
WISE EACH AND
EVERY DAY.

Breakfast:

Snack:

Lunch:

Snack:

Dinner:

Treat:

Exercise (optional):

Think Fit™

The Stubborn Fat Gone Shake

12 raw macadamia nuts

Shrimp Caesar Salad: Toss together 5 medium cooked shrimp, 2 cups shredded romaine, 5 cherry tomatoes, and 2 Tbsp. Caesar dressing.

2 slices salami spread with cream cheese

Dijon Chicken: Pan-fry 1 chicken breast, seasoned to taste and topped with 1 Tbsp. Dijon mustard. Serve with ¼ cup sautéed zucchini, seasoned to taste.

one glass red wine (15 Sugar Calories)

Today is a rest day.

Through reading these affirmations and messages on your weight-loss journey, you're growing more intuitive, inspired, and wise each day.

One benefit to this will be a newfound perspective on many things. For example, when you're invited to a party or a special event, you'll remember that your reason for attending is not the food. Instead, you enjoy the company of the people you're with and the experiences you're sharing.

At any party or event with friends, shift the focus from the food to the fun. While snacking is certainly part of the scene, instead of eyeing the next three platters you want to hit, pick three people you want to talk to. Your relationship with these old or new friends can be long-lasting. The relationship with those egg rolls or jalapeño poppers will most certainly be short-lived.

If you're going to a new place, rather than thinking about the restaurants you want to try, keep your mind on the experiences you'll have. For example, if you're going to the zoo and you love the elephants, it's easier to ignore the snack stands as you trek over to see them. When you go to an amusement park, try a thrilling ride you've never been on. You'll be sure to impress your kids.

Take a few minutes to think of other situations in which you can choose fun over food.

> *"I take the true definition of exercise to be labor without weariness."* — Samuel Johnson

WILLPOWER IS ONE OF MY SUPERPOWERS.

Breakfast:

Snack:

Lunch:

Snack:

Dinner:

Treat:

Exercise (optional):

Think Fit™

The Stubborn Fat Gone Shake

¼ cup sunflower seeds

Blue Chopped Salad: Toss together 2 cups shredded romaine, 4 slices chopped deli turkey, 1 chopped hard-boiled egg, 2 Tbsp. blue cheese crumbles, and 2 Tbsp. blue cheese dressing.

one hard-boiled egg

Grilled Flank Steak: Grill to desired doneness one 3-oz. flank steak, seasoned to taste. Serve with a side salad of 2 cups spinach, 5 sliced cherry tomatoes, 2 Tbsp. feta cheese, and a dressing of olive oil and vinegar.

one glass red wine (15 Sugar Calories)

Do a high-intensity interval training workout.

Simply put, willpower is having the strength to resist short-term temptations in order to reach long-term goals. Willpower is what allows you to pass on the breadbasket by keeping your eye on the prize.

Want some willpower? Pick up some weights. If you're planning on going out or meeting up with friends today, ask them to join you in a brisk walk or some form of exercise you enjoy. Moving your body triggers chemical messengers that boost your motivation, energy, and impulse control, so you'll be better armed for any occasion.

Multiple studies show that exercise boosts willpower. In a study conducted at Macquarie University in Sydney, Australia, scientists showed that when people engaged in an exercise program for two months, they did better on a lab measure of self-control than when they didn't exercise. Compared to the control phase in which they did not exercise, participants reported significant decreases in stress and emotional distress; lower consumption of alcohol, cigarettes, and caffeine; increases in healthy eating, emotional control, maintenance of household chores, attendance to commitments, and monitoring of spending; and an improvement in study habits. In other words, by regularly exercising their willpower with physical exercise, this carried over to stronger willpower in nearly all areas of their lives.

Think about the biggest challenges to your willpower and how you will overcome each one.

> *"Failing to plan is planning to fail."* — Alan Lakein

PRIOR PLANNING PREVENTS POOR PERFORMANCE.

Breakfast:

Snack:

Lunch:

Snack:

Dinner:

Treat:

Exercise:

Think Fit™

The Stubborn Fat Gone Shake

12 raw macadamia nuts

Tossed Italian Salad: Toss together ½ cup steamed, chopped cauliflower; ½ cup steamed, chopped broccoli; 2 Tbsp. chopped red bell pepper; 3 sliced chopped ham; 2 Tbsp. olive oil; and salt and pepper, to taste.

2 slices salami spread with cream cheese

Cheesy Turkey Burger: Top 1 grilled turkey burger patty with 1 slice provolone, 2 slices tomato, and 1 Tbsp. mustard. Serve on ¼ cup bed of arugula.

one glass red wine (15 Sugar Calories)

Today is a rest day.

Your best weight-loss tool is your brain. You can use it to succeed in any situation. For example, if you wake up already craving carbs, satisfy your body with a healthy serving of brown rice for breakfast or hearty, whole-grain bread at lunch so that the baked goods at the coffee shop are less tempting. Research shows that eating a small serving of healthy carbohydrates can boost your serotonin, which lowers further cravings for carbs, reduces your appetite, and boosts your impulse control.

Having delicious meals before going to a get-together or party will help you stick to your goals at the event, so that when you're faced with temptation, you don't succumb to a throw-in-the-towel mentality. So if you're going to an evening event, be sure to eat healthy fats, proteins, and vegetables early in your day. Don't go to the party starving, because that sets you up to overeat the wrong sorts of foods. Enjoy a healthy snack about an hour before the party so you can resist the hors d'oeuvres.

Think about your next social event and come up with three strategies you can do beforehand to prepare yourself.

"*Kindness in words creates confidence. Kindness in thinking creates profoundness. Kindness in giving creates love.*" — Lao-tzu

MY
KINDNESS
CAN HELP
ME STAY ON
TRACK.

Breakfast:

Snack:

Lunch:

Snack:

Dinner:

Treat:

Exercise (optional):

Think Fit™

The Stubborn Fat Gone Shake

¼ cup sunflower seeds

Shrimp Caesar Salad: Toss together 5 medium cooked shrimp, 2 cups shredded romaine, 5 cherry tomatoes, and 2 Tbsp. Caesar dressing.

one hard-boiled egg

Dijon Chicken: Pan-fry 1 chicken breast, seasoned to taste and topped with 1 Tbsp. Dijon mustard. Serve with ¼ cup sautéed zucchini, seasoned to taste.

one glass red wine (15 Sugar Calories)

Do a high-intensity interval training workout.

Today let's talk more about parties. If you're planning on going to an event, there's no reason to go empty-handed! Most hosts would welcome offers to bring food to share. For courtesy's sake, call ahead and politely offer to make a dish or appetizer. Then, once you've offered, be certain to bring it; the host is counting on you! This is also your opportunity to bring something healthy that you know you can eat. As a bonus, you'll get to share a favorite recipe with the other guests.

Here are a few examples for low- to no-sugar foods to bring:

- Celery with cream cheese and blue cheese. Just mix the two cheeses together and spread—delicious!

- Antipasto salad with Italian meats and cheeses. If you purchase this in a store, be sure to read the nutrition label.

- Gourmet olives. Many grocery stores now feature an "olive bar" with several different types of olives. Be sure to bring toothpicks or other items for serving.

- Deviled eggs. Easy to make and always a party favorite.

Now think about some of your favorite healthy recipes that you can take to parties.

"When we are no longer able to change a situation, we are challenged to change ourselves." — Viktor Frankl

I AM AT EASE IN ALL SOCIAL SITUATIONS AND INTERACTIONS.

Breakfast:

Snack:

Lunch:

Snack:

Dinner:

Treat:

Exercise (optional):

Think Fit™

The Stubborn Fat Gone Shake

12 raw macadamia nuts

Blue Chopped Salad: Toss together 2 cups shredded romaine, 4 slices chopped deli turkey, 1 chopped hard-boiled egg, 2 Tbsp. blue cheese crumbles, and 2 Tbsp. blue cheese dressing.

2 slices salami spread with cream cheese

Grilled Flank Steak: Grill to desired doneness one 3-oz. flank steak, seasoned to taste. Serve with a side salad of 2 cups spinach, 5 sliced cherry tomatoes, 2 Tbsp. feta cheese, and a dressing of olive oil and vinegar.

one glass red wine (15 Sugar Calories)

Today is a rest day.

Are you a nervous nibbler? Many people are. When you're uneasy, it's common to use eating to try to distract yourself from those feelings. In a social situation, it's a good bet that the food within reach isn't something that will help you meet your health and weight-loss goals.

I feel that the best way to combat nervous nibbling is to not get anxious in the first place! And one of the simplest ways to start feeling at ease is to simply *go easy* on yourself. Give yourself some slack for how you look and how you feel. If you haven't reached a health goal as quickly as you'd like, remind yourself of how hard you've been working on it; know that you'll get there in time. If you're feeling down about yourself, think about all of the wonderful qualities that you possess.

My wish for you is that you can read today's affirmation and truly feel it in your heart. Being at ease is such a wonderful thing. Imagine attending a party and not feeling nervous at all. Instead, you're perfectly comfortable. Wouldn't that be fabulous?

Take a deep breath and look around. There's a good chance that the person standing next to you is nervous, too. See, you have something in common! Smile and say hello.

Brainstorm some other ways that will help you feel at ease in social situations. What are some healthier habits that can take the place of your nervous nibbling?

> " *If you can't fly, run. If you can't run, walk. If you can't walk, crawl. But by all means, keep moving.* "
>
> — Martin Luther King, Jr.

I DO NOT LOOK BACK;
I AM NOT GOING THAT WAY.

TRACKER

Breakfast:

Snack:

Lunch:

Snack:

Dinner:

Treat:

Exercise (optional):

Think Fit™

The Stubborn Fat Gone Shake

¼ cup sunflower seeds

Tossed Italian Salad: Toss together ½ cup steamed, chopped cauliflower; ½ cup steamed, chopped broccoli; 2 Tbsp. chopped red bell pepper; 3 sliced chopped ham; 2 Tbsp. olive oil; and salt and pepper, to taste.

one hard-boiled egg

Cheesy Turkey Burger: Top 1 grilled turkey burger patty with 1 slice provolone, 2 slices tomato, and 1 Tbsp. mustard. Serve on ¼ cup bed of arugula.

one glass red wine (15 Sugar Calories)

Today is a rest day.

Today's message is powerfully short: Stop looking back. Why? Because looking back really doesn't do you any good. You can't change the past. It's over, for better or for worse. Yes, you can learn from what you've done and apply it to your life in the present. But what you shouldn't do is ruminate on your past. In other words, don't think about something again and again, as if your mind were stuck in a loop. In fact, another expression for ruminating is "chewing the cud," like a cow eating grass. Well, you surely don't want to do that!

If you continuously finding yourself obsessing about the past, develop ways to unstick your mind. It might be as simple as wearing a rubber band around your wrist and snapping it whenever you catch yourself dwelling. A simple change in your environment can also work to get your mind of its rut. For example, getting up and going for a walk or getting a drink of water can shift your thoughts out of its obsessive track.

Keep your eyes forward and stay focused on your goals. Always remind yourself of why you are doing all of this—for your future.

Take a few minutes to think of ways you can "unstick" your brain if you catch yourself chewing the cud.

13

focus on success

The Stubborn Fat Gone™ program offers a lot of opportunities for reflection, and this week is going to be filled with it. I like to say that just as you can't drive your car while staring in the rearview mirror, you can't get anywhere in life if your thoughts are fixated on the past. Everyone makes mistakes, but what sets winners apart is that they're able to learn from their mistakes and grow.

It's important to remember, however, that you also can't live your life fearfully anticipating what *might* happen in the future. Going back to my car analogy, it'd be like trying to drive with your vision focused several miles down the road, while ignoring your immediate surroundings.

You'd crash into a sign or bus along the way! Certainly it's beneficial to dream, set goals, and make plans. But the reality is, we all live in the present moment—not the past or the future. The present is when you make your choices, and your decisions today shape your future.

Sit still for a moment and clear your mind. What are you doing? Breathing! Every second of every day, you are bringing new air into your body. This presents an incredible opportunity because a dramatic, effective way to change your present —your reality—is to change your breathing. We'll get into that, and more, soon. Breathe easy; it's going to be a great week!

> " *In order to succeed, your desire for success should be greater than your fear of failure.* "
> — Bill Cosby

I CAN
HANDLE
THIS.
I CAN DO
ANYTHING I PUT
MY MIND TO.

Breakfast:

Snack:

Lunch:

Snack:

Dinner:

Treat:

Exercise (optional):

Think Fit™

The Stubborn Fat Gone Shake

¼ cup pecans

Bacon Caprese Stack: Alternate 3 slices fresh mozzarella, 3 slices tomato, 3 strips cooked bacon, and 3 basil leaves in a stack. Drizzle with 1 Tbsp. balsamic vinegar.

one string cheese

Seasoned Salmon Spinach Salad: Rub one 3-oz. salmon fillet with butter and season with fresh dill. Grill, then serve atop 2 cups spinach with olive-oil-and-vinegar dressing.

one glass red wine (15 Sugar Calories)

Do a high-intensity interval training workout.

As you begin the eighth week of this program, I bet your confidence has really grown. When you read today's affirmation, do you really own those words? *I know that you can do anything you put your mind to.* But the bigger question is, do *you* know it?

In my heart, I truly believe that I can do anything I put my mind to. Why? Because I have set many goals for myself, and I have met them. I've set long-term goals, short-term goals, and everything in between. I've set goals about every sort of thing you can imagine: nutrition, exercise, health, work, and relationships. When you accomplish a task you've set for yourself, you start to realize that you can do it. With each objective you meet, your confidence builds.

Take a few minutes right now to think about how you've done so far on your weight-loss journey. How close are you to your goals? How far do you still have to go? How do you feel at this very moment?

> "*A man of genius makes no mistakes. His errors are volitional and the portals to discovery.*" — James Joyce

EVERY MISTAKE
I MAKE IS A VALUABLE OPPORTUNITY TO LEARN.

Breakfast:

Snack:

Lunch:

Snack:

Dinner:

Treat:

Exercise (optional):

Think Fit™

The Stubborn Fat Gone Shake

¼ cup Brazil nuts

Crunchy Chicken Wraps: Sauté 3 oz. chopped chicken breast, 2 stalks finely chopped celery, ½ cup chopped scallions, ½ cup chopped water chestnuts, 2 Tbsp. sliced almonds, 2 Tbsp. soy sauce, and crushed red pepper to taste. Evenly divide cooked mixture between 8 romaine lettuce leaves, about 2 to 3 Tbsp. per leaf. Serve with a side of ½ cup mushrooms and 4 asparagus stalks sautéed with soy sauce.

celery sticks spread with cream cheese

Zucchini Puffs: In a bowl, mix 3 Tbsp. mayonnaise, 3 Tbsp. Parmesan cheese, 1 Tbsp. basil, and chopped garlic and lemon juice to taste. Spread mixture evenly over 2 sliced zucchini in a baking dish. Broil in oven for 1 or 2 minutes, until top is browned. Serve with a side salad of 1 cup spinach and 1 sliced tomato, dressed with lemon juice.

one glass red wine (15 Sugar Calories)

Today is a rest day.

Yesterday, as you reflected on your progress of the past seven weeks, did you also think about any mistakes you've made? Maybe you skipped exercising for a few days, you gave in to temptation at an ice-cream stand, or you couldn't resist the siren call of the drive-through. Take two minutes and list a few of your mistakes in your journal. As you write, heed the famous words of Alexander Pope, "To err is human; to forgive, divine."

Yes, you've made some mistakes. You're only human, after all. But just as you would forgive your spouse, your parents, your children, and your friends their mistakes, be divine enough to forgive yourself. Go back to your journal, and next to each mistake that you listed, I want you to write, "I forgive myself."

Here's the next step you can take for real growth: Think about what you can learn from those mistakes. If you find it difficult to follow through with exercise, perhaps you could partner with a friend to hold you accountable. Order a luscious cheese plate at a restaurant instead of ice cream. And keep Freebie snacks on hand so you never let yourself get so hungry you can't resist the words "Would you like fries with that?"

"Happy is the person who knows what to remember of the past, what to enjoy in the present, and what to plan for in the future." — Arnold H. Glasow

I WISELY LOOK FORWARD AND PLAN FOR THE FUTURE.

Breakfast:

Snack:

Lunch:

Snack:

Dinner:

Treat:

Exercise (optional):

Think Fit™

The Stubborn Fat Gone Shake

¼ cup pecans

Broccoli Cheese Soup: Bring 2 cups chicken broth to a simmer, add 3 cups chopped broccoli, and cook until tender. In a separate pan, gently heat 4 oz. cream cheese and ¾ cup cream on low, stirring often. Purée broccoli mixture in a blender, then blend in cream-cheese mixture. Makes 4 servings; garnish each bowl with shredded cheddar cheese.

one string cheese

Spicy Taco Salad: Sauté ¼ lb. ground beef with 1 tsp. chili powder, ½ tsp. onion powder, and 1 clove minced garlic. Add to a bowl of 2 cups chopped salad greens, 1 chopped tomato, ½ chopped bell pepper, ½ sliced avocado, 1 Tbsp. sour cream, and 2 Tbsp. chopped cilantro. Top with 2 lime wedges.

one glass red wine (15 Sugar Calories)

Do a high-intensity interval training workout.

While your goals should always be at the forefront of your thoughts, today let's do something more concrete with them—more planning than dreaming. Look back on the past weeks and learn from your successes. What has worked well for you? How can you capitalize and build on your successes as you plan your upcoming weeks?

If you've just begun eating breakfast, starting your days off on the right foot, how can you continue that? Maybe you can buy the groceries you need for a week's worth of breakfasts, then prep and portion everything out on Sunday.

Or maybe a win for you has been that you replaced late-night snacking with a healthier habit. If you do yoga, you could support that by buying a new yoga mat. Or maybe you started to knit to keep your hands busy and out of the cracker box. Treat yourself to some new yarns so running out won't be a problem.

Take a few minutes to think about your biggest wins and how to support them in the future.

> " *Respect your efforts, respect yourself. Self-respect leads to self-discipline. When you have both firmly under your belt, that's real power.* " — Clint Eastwood

I CARRY MYSELF WITH **SELF-RESPECT** AND SELF-LOVE.

Breakfast:

Snack:

Lunch:

Snack:

Dinner:

Treat:

Exercise (optional):

Think Fit™

The Stubborn Fat Gone Shake

¼ cup Brazil nuts

Bacon Caprese Stack: Alternate 3 slices fresh mozzarella, 3 slices tomato, 3 strips cooked bacon, and 3 basil leaves in a stack. Drizzle with 1 Tbsp. balsamic vinegar.

celery sticks spread with cream cheese

Seasoned Salmon Spinach Salad: Rub one 3-oz. salmon fillet with butter and season with fresh dill. Grill, then serve atop 2 cups spinach with olive-oil-and-vinegar dressing.

one glass red wine (15 Sugar Calories)

Today is a rest day.

A few weeks ago, we talked about how you can see a person's confidence in the air that someone has about him- or herself. It's important to note that the way you carry yourself also reveals how much you respect and love yourself.

Think on it now: how much *do* you respect and love yourself? It's true that many of us have unrealistically high expectations for ourselves, and then we're hard on ourselves when we fail to live up to them. But when you respect yourself, you respect your body, and then you do the kinds of things that you are doing now— eating well, exercising, reducing stress, and taking care of yourself.

To love yourself, you need to be kind to yourself. Pay attention to the positive attributes you have. Celebrate yourself—like how you love animals, or the kind things you've done for a stranger. When you take time to notice the little good things that you do, you can see them build into bigger patterns of self-love.

Take a few minutes today to think about all of the things you love about yourself.

> *"Trust yourself. You know more than you think you do."* — Benjamin Spock

I LET GO AND **TRUST** THAT ALL IS HAPPENING AS IT **SHOULD.**

TRACKER

Breakfast:

Snack:

Lunch:

Snack:

Dinner:

Treat:

Exercise (optional):

Think Fit™

The Stubborn Fat Gone Shake

¼ cup pecans

Crunchy Chicken Wraps: Sauté 3 oz. chopped chicken breast, 2 stalks finely chopped celery, ½ cup chopped scallions, ½ cup chopped water chestnuts, 2 Tbsp. sliced almonds, 2 Tbsp. soy sauce, and crushed red pepper to taste. Evenly divide cooked mixture between 8 romaine lettuce leaves, about 2 to 3 Tbsp. per leaf. Serve with a side of ½ cup mushrooms and 4 asparagus stalks sautéed with soy sauce.

one string cheese

Zucchini Puffs: In a bowl, mix 3 Tbsp. mayonnaise, 3 Tbsp. Parmesan cheese, 1 Tbsp. basil, and chopped garlic and lemon juice to taste. Spread mixture evenly over 2 sliced zucchini in a baking dish. Broil in oven for 1 or 2 minutes, until top is browned. Serve with a side salad of 1 cup spinach and 1 sliced tomato, dressed with lemon juice.

one glass red wine (15 Sugar Calories)

Do a high-intensity interval training workout.

Today I want you to focus on feeling safe and protected. Imagine that you are surrounded by a force field of good, positive energy. This doesn't mean that negative things can't happen, but it bolsters your resolve and strength to face these challenges. You are protected. No negative energy can penetrate your shield. Trust your ability to protect yourself, and go without fear into this day.

I know that it can be hard to feel safe and have faith that everything is going to be okay. One thing that helps me tremendously is deep breathing. Have you noticed that when you feel anxious and fearful, you breathe more shallowly? On the flip side, deep breathing can reduce your cortisol levels and be tremendously calming. The following is a simple breathing exercise provided by Andrew Weil, M.D.:

1.   Exhale completely through your mouth, making a whoosh sound.
2.   Close your mouth and inhale quietly through your nose to a mental count of four.
3.   Hold your breath for a count of seven.
4.   Exhale completely through your mouth to a count of eight, making a whoosh sound.
5.   This is one breath cycle. Now repeat steps 2 through 4 three more times for a total of four breaths.

Think about the ways in which you are already safe and protected.

> ## "I always say shopping is cheaper than a psychiatrist."
> — Tammy Faye Bakker Messner

I AM
SAVVY
AND
SMART!

TRACKER

Breakfast:

Snack:

Lunch:

Snack:

Dinner:

Treat:

Exercise (optional):

Think Fit™

The Stubborn Fat Gone Shake

¼ cup Brazil nuts

Broccoli Cheese Soup: Bring 2 cups chicken broth to a simmer, add 3 cups chopped broccoli, and cook until tender. In a separate pan, gently heat 4 oz. cream cheese and ¾ cup cream on low, stirring often. Purée broccoli mixture in a blender, then blend in cream-cheese mixture. Makes 4 servings; garnish each bowl with shredded cheddar cheese.

celery sticks spread with cream cheese

Spicy Taco Salad: Sauté ¼ lb. ground beef with 1 tsp. chili powder, ½ tsp. onion powder, and 1 clove minced garlic. Add to a bowl of 2 cups chopped salad greens, 1 chopped tomato, ½ chopped bell pepper, ½ sliced avocado, 1 Tbsp. sour cream, and 2 Tbsp. chopped cilantro. Top with 2 lime wedges.

one glass red wine (15 Sugar Calories)

Today is a rest day.

You have to eat, and to do so, you have to shop. Unfortunately, the grocery store can be quite the minefield of challenges for people trying to improve their nutrition and get healthy.

Keep in mind these shopping tips: Never go to the store while hungry; you're more likely to make good decisions if you shop after you've eaten. You can also organize your shopping list to follow the map of the grocery store. Most stores are set up so that you have to walk past all sorts of temptations before you get to the foods you need. The healthiest foods tend to be on the outer aisles, with produce at the front and meats, dairy, and eggs along the back. You can get most items you need from these outer aisles, and avoid the center of the store where most processed foods are shelved. Remember: the more you stick to the perimeter, the better. If you shop in this way, keeping to your list of healthy foods and minimizing your exposure to whatever might ring the craving bell, you'll save time and money!

Think about some other ways you can set yourself up for success when shopping for healthy foods, and share them with your friends.

"*Accept the challenges so that you may feel the exhilaration of victory.*"

— General George S. Patton

I TAKE ON NEW CHALLENGES WITH CONFIDENCE, SKILL, AND EASE.

Breakfast:

Snack:

Lunch:

Snack:

Dinner:

Treat:

Exercise (optional):

Think Fit™

The Stubborn Fat Gone Shake

¼ cup pecans

Bacon Caprese Stack: Alternate 3 slices fresh mozzarella, 3 slices tomato, 3 strips cooked bacon, and 3 basil leaves in a stack. Drizzle with 1 Tbsp. balsamic vinegar.

one string cheese

Seasoned Salmon Spinach Salad: Rub one 3-oz. salmon fillet with butter and season with fresh dill. Grill, then serve atop 2 cups spinach with olive-oil-and-vinegar dressing.

one glass red wine (15 Sugar Calories)

Today is a rest day.

Over the past few weeks, did you discover any surprising weight-loss challenges? Today we'll continue to talk about a place that's a minefield for many: the grocery store!

Are the Girl Scouts stalking the entrance? Know this: the cookies just aren't worth it. One serving of Samoas (two cookies) has 72 Sugar Calories, and a serving of Thin Mints (four cookies) comes out to 88 Sugar Calories. A better way to offer support without giving in to the temptation is to give a donation. Or you can buy a box of cookies and give it to the girls who are selling them.

Is your store "generously" handing out samples? They probably aren't offering steamed broccoli or grilled tilapia! Smile and pass on the crackers, dips, and candies. Better yet, keep yourself occupied by chewing a stick of gum while you're shopping.

Do you shop with your kids? When they ask you to "c'mere!" and see the newest candy or buy them a doughnut from the case, you don't have to give in. Keep the kids busy helping you cross items off of your list or pulling coupons from your stash. If they're old enough, allow them to pick up items for you a few aisles over. Remember to reward them with something other than food, such as a trip to the library or park.

Take a few minutes to reflect on some of the weight-loss challenges you've discovered and the clever ways you were able to overcome them.

14

let your body *move*

After all these weeks of effort, you've really started to transform your body. I bet that you also have lots more energy to boot! With all these changes, your body will naturally crave more movement. Keeping your muscles strong and toned improves your cardiovascular health, and having more muscle mass keeps your metabolism high, which makes it even easier to keep the fat off!

This week, I'm going to share with you a few of my secret tips for toning your body. I'd like to encourage you to add some exercise into your daily life for strength and general health. A certain kind of joy settles into your spirit and fills your being with buzzing energy and peaceful ease. . . . That's the kind of exercise I want for you!

"Winning is only half of it. Having fun is the other half." — Bum Phillips

I HAVE COME SO FAR, AND I KNOW I CAN DO EVEN MORE!

TRACKER

Breakfast:

Snack:

Lunch:

Snack:

Dinner:

Treat:

Exercise (optional):

Think Fit™

The Stubborn Fat Gone Shake

¼ cup almonds

Spinach Chicken Salad: Combine 1 sliced cooked chicken breast, 1 minced celery stalk, ¼ cup chopped almonds, 2 Tbsp. sour cream, 2 Tbsp. mayonnaise, 2 tsp. lemon juice, 2 Tbsp. Italian seasoning, and salt and pepper to taste. Toss together with 1½ cups spinach.

one hard-boiled egg

Signature Steak: Sauté ½ cup chopped onion, 1 chopped bell pepper, and 1 Tbsp. thyme. Reduce heat to low, add 2 Tbsp. dry red wine, and simmer a few minutes. Plate mixture with 3 oz. grilled flank steak and top with 2 Tbsp. crumbled goat cheese.

one glass red wine (15 Sugar Calories)

Do a high-intensity interval training workout.

Welcome to the beginning of Week 9. Congratulations on all of your progress and all of your success—you've come so far!

This is a fabulous time to offer yourself a really great treat. Take some time to think about a reward that will do two important things. First, it should make you feel like you have truly accomplished something, because you have. Second, it should motivate and inspire you to keep up the great work for the rest of this program.

You might be wondering if you can reward yourself with food. My answer is, "Yes, but . . ." It's okay to enjoy a healthful meal or snack, perhaps going out to a fine restaurant as your reward. Just know that eating a bag of chips or a box of cookies is not rewarding at all in the long run.

For me, the best rewards are spending time with my sons, enjoying an espresso with friends, pausing to watch the sunset on a beach, and going on vacation to see my extended family.

Think about what your reward will be and make a plan for when and how to enjoy it.

> *"Physical fitness is not only one of the most important keys to a healthy body; it is the basis of dynamic and creative intellectual activity."* — John F. Kennedy

I MAKE TIME TO EXERCISE BECAUSE I AM WORTH IT!

Breakfast:

Snack:

Lunch:

Snack:

Dinner:

Treat:

Exercise (optional):

Think Fit™

The Stubborn Fat Gone Shake

one string cheese

Bunless Burger: Use lettuce to wrap 1 cooked hamburger patty with ¼ sliced avocado, 5 slices cucumber, and mustard to taste.

cucumber slices with feta cheese

Lemon Grilled Salmon: Grill 1 salmon fillet, seasoned with lemon juice, salt, and pepper to taste. Serve with ½ cup steamed broccoli, seasoned to taste.

one glass red wine (15 Sugar Calories)

Today is a rest day.

For good health and weight loss, eating well and movement go together like chocolate and peanut butter. Exercise can help you in so many ways. One of the most important is that it reduces your body's levels of cortisol, the stress hormone that causes you to store fat.

Don't stress about how you'll fit more physical activity into your calendar. Things such as going on a walk, taking the kids to the park, vigorous housework, and gardening can all be added in at any time. Just throw on a headset with some great music and enjoy whatever you're doing!

Research shows that physical activity in the morning can help raise your metabolism for the rest of the day. It launches you into your day with a positive mind-set, and you'll also feel energized afterward and more awake. So those minutes you give up to get active will actually give you back more hours in your day.

Pick the most convenient time for you to care for your body with movement. Take a few minutes to think about ways to incorporate fitness into your life.

"Those who think they have not time for bodily exercise will sooner or later have to find time for illness." — Edward Stanley

I TAKE JOY IN IMPROVING MYSELF.

TRACKER

Breakfast:

Snack:

Lunch:

Snack:

Dinner:

Treat:

Exercise (optional):

Think Fit™

The Stubborn Fat Gone Shake

¼ cup almonds

Chicken Sauté: Sauté 1 sliced chicken breast with ¼ cup red bell peppers, ¼ cup chopped onion, and ½ cup broccoli. Salt and pepper to taste.

one hard-boiled egg

Mushroom Pork Chop: Sauté 1 pork chop and top with ½ cup sautéed mushrooms. Serve with a side of ½ cup steamed broccoli. Season all with salt and pepper, to taste.

one glass red wine (15 Sugar Calories)

Do a high-intensity interval training workout.

I know you're busy; I am, too. It seems that you run out of "today" before you run out of to-dos. It can be hard to find the time to exercise as your days fly by. Want the secret that makes it easier to stay active? Make it fun. You'll always find ways to fit fun into your day.

Take a few minutes today to think about activities that you think are enjoyable. For example, I recently went snorkeling, and I'll often play with my kids on the beach or take them on a hike. If you like to plan outings with your kids, rather than going to a movie or other passive event, go to a trampoline or inflatable bounce place. Don't just watch your kids, bounce right along with them. You'll be amazed by how much fun it is.

> "*Discipline is the bridge between goals and accomplishment.*"
>
> — Jim Rohn

I HAVE THE **POWER** AND **WISDOM** TO HAVE THE BEST, HEALTHIEST DAY YET.

TRACKER

Breakfast:

Snack:

Lunch:

Snack:

Dinner:

Treat:

Exercise (optional):

Think Fit™

The Stubborn Fat Gone Shake

one string cheese

Spinach Chicken Salad: Combine 1 sliced cooked chicken breast, 1 minced celery stalk, ¼ cup chopped almonds, 2 Tbsp. sour cream, 2 Tbsp. mayonnaise, 2 tsp. lemon juice, 2 Tbsp. Italian seasoning, and salt and pepper to taste. Toss together with 1½ cups spinach.

cucumber slices with feta cheese

Signature Steak: Sauté ½ cup chopped onion, 1 chopped bell pepper, and 1 Tbsp. thyme. Reduce heat to low, add 2 Tbsp. dry red wine, and simmer a few minutes. Plate mixture with 3 oz. grilled flank steak and top with 2 Tbsp. crumbled goat cheese.

one glass red wine (15 Sugar Calories)

Today is a rest day.

Discipline and strength are a formidable combination. To stick to your plan and to meet your goals, you'll need a healthy dose of each.

One way that you can gauge discipline and strength is by looking at a person's posture. Take a second to think about how you are sitting. Are you lounging on the couch reading this book? Are your shoulders slouched, making your back form a C? If so, you're cheating your body! Furthermore, you're not projecting a disciplined, strong image to the world—or even to yourself.

Today's exercise is to work on your posture. (Wouldn't your mother be proud?) You may be surprised by how these tips can even boost your confidence. They'll also open up your breathing passages and increase your blood flow. Here are some key posture points:

- Sit up straight.
- Walk tall with your shoulders back, which puts a small curve in your back.
- When you're walking, pull in your core muscles, and hold tight.

Give these posture pointers a try. Note which worked best for you, and practice them again and again until they become natural.

"Walking is the best possible exercise. Habituate yourself to walk very far." — Thomas Jefferson

I WAS
MADE
TO BE
MOBILE!

Breakfast:

Snack:

Lunch:

Snack:

Dinner:

Treat:

Exercise (optional):

Think Fit™

The Stubborn Fat Gone Shake

¼ cup almonds

Bunless Burger: Use lettuce to wrap 1 cooked hamburger patty with ¼ sliced avocado, 5 slices cucumber, and mustard to taste.

one hard-boiled egg

Lemon Grilled Salmon: Grill 1 salmon fillet, seasoned with lemon juice, salt, and pepper to taste. Serve with ½ cup steamed broccoli, seasoned to taste.

one glass red wine (15 Sugar Calories)

Do a high-intensity interval training workout.

If you need some help with motivation today, consider this your wake-up call. Take a walk!

When you go for a walk for your body, your mind will thank you for it. This simple act comes with so many health benefits. Experts say that walking can help you:

- Maintain a healthy weight.
- Prevent or manage health conditions, such as heart disease, high blood pressure, and diabetes.
- Strengthen your bones.
- Lift your mood.
- Improve your balance and coordination.

When it comes to walking, you can't have too much of a good thing. The faster, farther, and more frequently you walk, the greater the benefits you'll enjoy. Go outside and appreciate the scenery—enjoy the flowers, watch the trees move in the wind, and take note of clouds on the horizon. When you take in the natural delights of the outdoors, you boost your levels of serotonin, the feel-good hormone, which is always a good thing. If you don't like to walk by yourself, encourage your spouse, children, or friends to join you. You can motivate each other toward greater health.

Take a few minutes to think about the reasons you enjoy walking and ways you can enjoy it more.

> " *Success is due to our stretching to the challenges of life. Failure comes when we shrink from them.* " — John C. Maxwell

I AM
STRETCHING
AND
GROWING
EVERY DAY.

Breakfast:

Snack:

Lunch:

Snack:

Dinner:

Treat:

Exercise (optional):

Think Fit™

The Stubborn Fat Gone Shake

one string cheese

Chicken Sauté: Sauté 1 sliced chicken breast with ¼ cup red bell peppers, ¼ cup chopped onion, and ½ cup broccoli. Salt and pepper to taste.

cucumber slices with feta cheese

Mushroom Pork Chop: Sauté 1 pork chop and top with ½ cup sautéed mushrooms. Serve with a side of ½ cup steamed broccoli. Season all with salt and pepper, to taste.

one glass red wine (15 Sugar Calories)

Today is a rest day.

As you read each day's affirmations and reflect on the message, you are mentally stretching and growing. That's great, but with growing often comes some pains! So today, let's combat those pains with some actual, physical stretching.

Your head probably weighs about ten pounds; your worries weigh a whole lot more. Most of us hold stress in our necks and shoulder muscles, which can lead to pain and stiffness. Stretching your neck can relieve that stress-induced tension. Take a minute for yourself and gently stretch your neck out with the following exercise.

1. Sit up straight in a chair with your shoulders aligned over your hips. Tuck your chin and tilt your head down to stretch the back of your neck. Hold this position for up to 20 seconds, then relax and return your head to the neutral position.
2. Tilt your chin toward the ceiling to stretch the front of your neck. Hold for up to 20 seconds, then relax and return your head to the neutral position.
3. Tilt your right ear to your right shoulder, and hold for up to 20 seconds. Then tilt your left ear to your left shoulder, and hold for up to 20 seconds. Return to the neutral position, and relax.
4. Repeat the head tilts and extension a few times on all sides.
5. Finally, take a deep, cleansing breath, and relax.

Take a few minutes to think about the ways you are stretching and growing in all areas of your life.

God grant me the serenity to accept the things I cannot change, the courage to change the things I can, and the wisdom to know the difference.

— Reinhold Niebuhr

I AM FULL OF SERENITY AND COURAGE.

Breakfast:

Snack:

Lunch:

Snack:

Dinner:

Treat:

Exercise (optional):

Think Fit™

The Stubborn Fat Gone Shake

¼ cup almonds

Spinach Chicken Salad: Combine 1 sliced cooked chicken breast, 1 minced celery stalk, ¼ cup chopped almonds, 2 Tbsp. sour cream, 2 Tbsp. mayonnaise, 2 tsp. lemon juice, 2 Tbsp. Italian seasoning, and salt and pepper to taste. Toss together with 1½ cups spinach.

one hard-boiled egg

Signature Steak: Sauté ½ cup chopped onion, 1 chopped bell pepper, and 1 Tbsp. thyme. Reduce heat to low, add 2 Tbsp. dry red wine, and simmer a few minutes. Plate mixture with 3 oz. grilled flank steak and top with 2 Tbsp. crumbled goat cheese.

one glass red wine (15 Sugar Calories)

Today is a rest day.

After working this week on physical activity, posture, and stretching, I bet you feel both serene and courageous. Do these two words seem almost incompatible? Keep in mind, however, that exercise is amazing for making us feel both calm and brave at the same time. According to doctors at the Mayo Clinic, exercise eases depression and anxiety by releasing feel-good brain chemicals. It also boosts your body temperature, which can have a calming effect, along with boosting your confidence, which makes you feel braver.

What kind of exercise is best? Walking, lifting weights, and spinning are all wonderful. But the best activity is whatever motivates you to move—to get up off the couch and stick to it.

With advice and encouragement from me, your support circle, and yourself, you now *know* that you can do anything you put your mind to. You have done so well, so make sure to treat yourself to something special today to reward your hard work.

Take a few minutes to think about your favorite exercises and how they make your body and mind feel.

15

understand the path of indulgence

It's time to celebrate! I bet if I polled a large group of people about what they consider indulgences, the majority of them would be about food. Is that true for you? I challenge you to expand your thinking and broaden your definition of what the word can encompass.

You can enjoy treats, because you deserve them. Your life can overflow with abundance. We're all wired to crave indulgence. We seek out things that make us feel good, and when something makes us feel good, we want more, and more, and more. You can use Think Fit™ strategies to identify and enjoy the indulgences that support your health rather than those that undermine it. You have the power to think the thoughts and to make the choices that will keep you on the right path to weight loss and great health.

One of the things we're going to talk about this week as an indulgence might surprise you. Though if you're a parent and remember those early months with a fussy infant, it might not be a shock at all—it's sleep! Great sleep is the ultimate treat. Give yourself a break today!

"We are all deserving of love." — Sandra Bullock

I AM A WORTHWHILE PERSON WHO DESERVES LOVE AND RESPECT.

Breakfast:

Snack:

Lunch:

Snack:

Dinner:

Treat:

Exercise (optional):

Think Fit™

The Stubborn Fat Gone Shake

celery sticks with almond butter

Chopped Salad: Top 2 cups chopped romaine lettuce with 1 chopped hard-boiled egg, ¼ diced avocado, ¼ cup diced tomatoes, 1 thinly sliced green onion, and ½ cup diced turkey breast. Dress with olive oil and vinegar.

¼ cup mixed nuts

Grilled Tilapia: Grill 1 tilapia fillet, seasoned to taste with lemon juice, salt, and pepper. Serve with ½ cup sautéed zucchini.

one glass red wine (15 Sugar Calories)

Do a high-intensity interval training workout.

R-E-S-P-E-C-T, let's find out what it means to you. Does it mean someone listening to you? Responding to you in a positive way? Showing appreciation for you? Before you can recognize yourself as being worthy of indulgences, you must first see yourself as deserving of respect.

Take a couple minutes and think about the names of three people you really respect. Now think about the names of three people who really respect you. There's a good chance you've never taken the time to think about that. Are there any people who you feel don't respect you?

To have someone's respect is one thing, but to have respect and love is something quite different. While they are so intertwined that some might say, "love is respect," it's possible to respect someone without loving them. Think of a grade-school teacher, a policeman who pulls you over for speeding, or an Army drill sergeant. On the flip side, is it possible to love someone without respecting them? I don't think so. I think that love is built upon a strong foundation of many things, one of which is respect.

Take a few minutes now to think about how you are deserving of both love and respect—from your spouse, your parents, your children, and your friends.

> " *Believe me, the reward is not so great without the struggle.* "
> —Wilma Rudolph

I AM
WORTHY
OF
INDULGENCE.

Breakfast:

Snack:

Lunch:

Snack:

Dinner:

Treat:

Exercise (optional):

Think Fit™

The Stubborn Fat Gone Shake

2 slices deli meat

Asian Chicken Salad: For dressing, combine 2 Tbsp. mayonnaise, 1 tsp. soy sauce, and ¼ tsp. lemon juice. In a separate bowl, combine 2 cups mixed greens with ½ cup diced, cooked chicken breast; ¼ cup chopped celery; and 2 Tbsp. chopped water chestnuts. Salt and pepper to taste.

2 slices cheddar cheese

Grilled Kebab: Briefly soak a wooden skewer in water. Alternate three 1" cubes of top sirloin, 3 slices red bell pepper, and 3 slices mushroom onto skewer. Season with salt and pepper, then grill over medium heat, turning halfway through cooking.

one glass red wine (15 Sugar Calories)

Today is a rest day.

What is your view of indulgences? You might think of the word in terms of delicious things to eat, or you might have been told that you can't reward yourself with food treats. On this program, as you can see from the Food Lists in Chapter 3, you can certainly indulge occasionally in foods such as chocolate and wine. However, I want to encourage you to expand your definition of *indulgence* to include any activity or expression of self-care. When you take care of and treat yourself, everyone benefits.

Think of the standard instructions given on an airplane. You are always told to put your oxygen mask on yourself first before helping others. By taking some "me time," you achieve a centered, calm sense of peace, and you carry this energy with you as you interact with your children, your spouse, friends, family, and co-workers.

One thing I love to do in my "me time" is listen to my favorite music. Have you ever noticed how music can instantly change your mood? Your favorite song comes on the radio, and you brighten up. You hear the strains of a soothing lullaby, and you relax. Studies show that listening to music can lower your cortisol levels. What's the soundtrack to *your* life? I encourage you to listen to it often.

Take a few minutes today to brainstorm non-food treats and indulgences that you enjoy.

TRACKER

"Abundance is not something we acquire. It is something we tune in to." — Wayne W. Dyer

MY LIFE OVERFLOWS WITH ABUNDANCE; MY SOUL OVERFLOWS WITH JOY.

Breakfast:

Snack:

Lunch:

Snack:

Dinner:

Treat:

Exercise (optional):

Think Fit™

The Stubborn Fat Gone Shake

celery sticks with almond butter

Lemon Chicken with Roasted Veggies: Preheat oven to 400° F. Season 1 chicken breast with 1 Tbsp. lemon juice, ½ Tbsp. olive oil, and salt and pepper. Place in greased baking dish and cook for 40 to 45 minutes. Serve with a side of ¼ cup sautéed mushrooms and ½ cup sautéed broccoli, seasoned to taste.

¼ cup mixed nuts

Portobello Pizzas: Preheat oven to 450° F. Grill 2 portobello mushrooms on both sides. Scoop out black fins and fill each mushroom with 1 Tbsp. pesto, shredded mozzarella cheese, black olives, and chopped cooked bacon. Sprinkle with Parmesan cheese and place in oven for 5 minutes.

one glass red wine (15 Sugar Calories)

Do a high-intensity interval training workout.

At a very basic level, our brains are wired so that when something feels good, we want it again and again. We're motivated by rewards, which can include food, sex, and social interactions. They activate a pathway that tells you to repeat what you just did to get more. This is the reason that weight-loss programs based on deprivation fail. You just can't stick with it. It's human nature to want what you can't have.

On this program, I encourage you to enjoy a full life, filled with everyday treats—in fact, a life filled with abundance. That's the kind of healthy plan that you'll stick with. Here are some healthy treat options:

- Red wine, 5 oz.: 15 Sugar Calories
- White wine, 5 oz.: 15 Sugar Calories
- Popcorn, air popped, 1 cup: 25 Sugar Calories
- Green & Black's 85% Dark Chocolate, 6 pieces: 30 Sugar Calories
- Barlean's Chocolate Raspberry Swirl: Freebie
- Apricot, 1: 16 Sugar Calories
- Trail mix, 1 oz.: 45 Sugar Calories
- Almond butter topped with whipped cream: Freebie

Write down some of your favorite healthy treats. What are some easy ways to keep them on hand?

> *"Sleep is that golden chain that ties health and our bodies together."* —Thomas Dekker

I DESERVE A
BREAK
TODAY.

Breakfast:

Snack:

Lunch:

Snack:

Dinner:

Treat:

Exercise (optional):

Think Fit™

The Stubborn Fat Gone Shake

2 slices deli meat

Chopped Salad: Top 2 cups chopped romaine lettuce with 1 chopped hard-boiled egg, ¼ diced avocado, ¼ cup diced tomatoes, 1 thinly sliced green onion, and ½ cup diced turkey breast. Dress with olive oil and vinegar.

2 slices cheddar cheese

Grilled Tilapia: Grill 1 tilapia fillet, seasoned to taste with lemon juice, salt, and pepper. Serve with ½ cup sautéed zucchini.

one glass red wine (15 Sugar Calories)

Today is a rest day.

I might not agree with much that fast-food chains do, but I do enjoy that famous slogan: You deserve a break today!

You can sleep your way to health and beauty. As simple as that may sound, it is estimated that up to 40 million Americans suffer from one of more than 70 different sleep disorders. Sleep directly affects your health, mood, and appearance, so you would think we would get more of this essential activity. However, it's common for many Americans to sleep 6 hours or less a night.

Furthermore, sleep is crucial for weight loss. Sometimes the best thing you can do is just to sleep more. It allows your central nervous system to relax, and when you're not as stressed, your body is able to release fat.

Your goal should be to get eight hours of "quality" sleep each night. To that end, these are a few of my favorite tips:

- *Schedule your sleep.* Calculate what time you would need to get into bed, factoring in the time it takes you to actually fall asleep, in order to get eight hours of sleep.
- *Exercise.* It aids weight loss, it's beneficial for your overall health, and studies have shown that people who exercise regularly get better sleep.
- *Avoid midafternoon caffeine.* Caffeine can take hours to wear off, so consumption in the afternoon can affect the restfulness of your sleep.

Take a few minutes to remember some happy dreams. Writing them down in your journal each morning can be a great way to keep track of them. Sweet dreams, my friend!

"When I was around 18, I looked in the mirror and said, 'You're either going to love yourself or hate yourself.' And I decided to love myself. That changed a lot of things." — Queen Latifah

I **BELIEVE** IN **MYSELF** ENTIRELY. I AM STRONG AND CAPABLE.

TRACKER

Breakfast:

Snack:

Lunch:

Snack:

Dinner:

Treat:

Exercise (optional):

Think Fit™

The Stubborn Fat Gone Shake

celery sticks with almond butter

Asian Chicken Salad: For dressing, combine 2 Tbsp. mayonnaise, 1 tsp. soy sauce, and ¼ tsp. lemon juice. In a separate bowl, combine 2 cups mixed greens with ½ cup diced, cooked chicken breast; ¼ cup chopped celery; and 2 Tbsp. chopped water chestnuts. Salt and pepper to taste.

¼ cup mixed nuts

Grilled Kebab: Briefly soak a wooden skewer in water. Alternate three 1" cubes of top sirloin, 3 slices red bell pepper, and 3 slices mushroom onto skewer. Season with salt and pepper, then grill over medium heat, turning halfway through cooking.

one glass red wine (15 Sugar Calories)

Do a high-intensity interval training workout.

Take a good look in the mirror. Are you seeing your biggest supporter, or are you facing your worst saboteur? When you look at yourself, do you focus on your best traits and smile? Or do you home in on the places that could use improvement and scowl?

Think about the words you say to yourself. Do you tell yourself things like, "You're too fat," "You will never be anything," and "That outfit makes you look hideous"? Anyone would be crushed to hear somebody say those hurtful words to them. I doubt you would ever say those things to your friend, your spouse, your parent, or your children. Why would you say them to yourself?

It's bad enough when others say these things, yet many of us are our own worst critics. Talking to ourselves like this is purely negative. Promise that you will no longer be so down on yourself. It's time to indulge yourself with supportive, loving self-talk. What would you want to hear or be pleased to have somebody compliment you on?

Think about some of the sabotaging thoughts you tend to tell yourself. Write down some daily affirmations that you can replace them with.

> "*A wise woman recognizes when her life is out of balance and summons the courage to act to correct it. A wise woman knows the meaning of true generosity. A wise woman knows happiness is the reward for a life lived in harmony, with courage and grace.*"
>
> — Suze Orman

I TRUST MYSELF TO LIVE MY LIFE WITH WISDOM AND GRACE.

TRACKER

Breakfast:

Snack:

Lunch:

Snack:

Dinner:

Treat:

Exercise (optional):

Think Fit™

The Stubborn Fat Gone Shake

2 slices deli meat

Lemon Chicken with Roasted Veggies: Preheat oven to 400° F. Season 1 chicken breast with 1 Tbsp. lemon juice, ½ Tbsp. olive oil, and salt and pepper. Place in greased baking dish and cook for 40 to 45 minutes. Serve with a side of ¼ cup sautéed mushrooms and ½ cup sautéed broccoli, seasoned to taste.

2 slices cheddar cheese

Portobello Pizzas: Preheat oven to 450° F. Grill 2 portobello mushrooms on both sides. Scoop out black fins and fill each mushroom with 1 Tbsp. pesto, shredded mozzarella cheese, black olives, and chopped cooked bacon. Sprinkle with Parmesan cheese and place in oven for 5 minutes.

one glass red wine (15 Sugar Calories)

Today is a rest day.

I love the word *grace.* It makes me think of my mother—a strong, elegant woman. My mother's grace springs from her inner strength and wisdom.

To find your grace, you need to tap into that strong, calm place within you. One way to center yourself is to indulge in a massage! Getting a massage can be much more than just a pleasurable treat. It's a fantastic way to relieve anxiety. You may be all too familiar with that tight feeling in your muscles you get when the stress piles up—you feel all tied into knots. A good massage therapist can help your body release that tension and trigger your brain to release natural painkillers and endorphins, which have a euphoric effect. Massage therapy also boosts your immune system and helps your body's lymphatic system drain toxins.

I recommend that you incorporate regular massages into your self-care regimen. You won't be sorry! Get a recommendation for a therapist and make an appointment. Reflect on why you deserve this gift.

> **"The greatest weapon against stress is our ability to choose one thought over another."** — William James

I CAN STRESS **LESS.**

Breakfast:

Snack:

Lunch:

Snack:

Dinner:

Treat:

Exercise (optional):

Think Fit™

The Stubborn Fat Gone Shake

celery sticks with almond butter

Chopped Salad: Top 2 cups chopped romaine lettuce with 1 chopped hard-boiled egg, ¼ diced avocado, ¼ cup diced tomatoes, 1 thinly sliced green onion, and ½ cup diced turkey breast. Dress with olive oil and vinegar.

¼ cup mixed nuts

Grilled Tilapia: Grill 1 tilapia fillet, seasoned to taste with lemon juice, salt, and pepper. Serve with ½ cup sautéed zucchini.

one glass red wine (15 Sugar Calories)

Today is a rest day.

Stress is universal; it's the great equalizer. You really can't avoid it, you certainly can't cure it, but you *can* learn how to manage it.

The struggles of stress and weight feed off each other in a vicious circle—like two kids hopped up on sugar on a playground, each magnifying the other. When you're stressed, you probably eat more, and your weight causes you further stress!

Stress is a mental and physical reaction we have to events that disrupt our personal balance in some way, and it can wreak havoc on your health if you're not careful. Before you run to the psychiatrist for help, I recommend that you try a more natural solution. Certain herbs have been used for centuries to help ease the effects of stress. Here are a few that I suggest. Consult with your doctor before taking any of these, as herbs may have adverse interactions with medications or health conditions.

- *Valerian:* Traditionally used to treat mild anxiety, valerian is usually taken about an hour before bedtime. It's a great sleep aid if stress keeps you awake at night.
- *Saint-John's-wort:* It's been used for centuries in many countries to reduce anxiety and to treat depression.
- *Chamomile:* Most often found in tea form, I usually have some after dinner because it aids in digestion and helps me fall asleep.

Take a few minutes to think of natural ways to help you stress less.

16

see a brand-new *you!*

I find the description *brand-new* to be very interesting. Let's riff off the word *brand* for a second. When I think of a brand, I think of a company, like Levi's. And when I think of Levi's, I think of the labels on the back of their jeans. And when I think about labels, I think about the many labels we assign to ourselves. Sadly, not all the labels we give ourselves are as nice or as innocuous as those little leather ones affixed to our jeans.

A label is any word you use to describe yourself, and it truly establishes how you see yourself. Whether you are conscious of it or not, you are continually perpetuating a certain vision of who you are based on these words. Do you call yourself fat? Lazy? Unhappy? Weak? Sometimes we slap labels on ourselves that we would never be cruel enough to call other people. We can be our own worst critics.

This week, you're going to think a lot about the way that you see and talk about yourself. I'm so excited for you to meet the new you!

> " *Be all you can be.* "
>
> — Former slogan of the U.S. Army

I AM THE
BEST
I HAVE
EVER BEEN.

TRACKER

Breakfast:

Snack:

Lunch:

Snack:

Dinner:

Treat:

Exercise (optional):

Think Fit™

The Stubborn Fat Gone Shake

¼ cup sunflower seeds

Tossed Italian Salad: Toss together ½ cup steamed, chopped cauliflower; ½ cup steamed, chopped broccoli; 2 Tbsp. chopped red bell pepper; 3 sliced chopped ham; 2 Tbsp. olive oil; and salt and pepper, to taste.

one hard-boiled egg

Cheesy Turkey Burger: Top 1 grilled turkey burger patty with 1 slice provolone, 2 slices tomato, and 1 Tbsp. mustard. Serve on ¼ cup bed of arugula.

one glass red wine (15 Sugar Calories)

Do a high-intensity interval training workout.

Repeat today's affirmation to yourself today and, more important, believe it. After all your hard work, you *are* the best you've ever been. You dug deep, committed fully, and changed your life. No one could ask for—or do—more. You are committed to your health, and that is an amazing accomplishment. Keep it up!

As we've discussed, a label is any word you use to describe yourself. So can you accept the label of "the best"? If that's a little difficult, try the following activity for reinventing your identity.

Think about all of the negative names you have for yourself, even the ones that are incredibly hurtful. In your mind, pick up all of these labels, crumple them up, and toss them right in the trash! Now see a clean, fresh piece of paper in your head. Think of your new "power" label—a word that can empower you to outstanding levels of confidence. Store it in the files of your brain. Think about that phrase every day and repeat it in your head, especially whenever you find yourself trying to dig up one of those old, negative names.

Take a few minutes and write down at least ten new, positive labels for yourself.

"*The more you like yourself, the less you are like anyone else, which makes you unique.*" — Walt Disney

I AM COMFORTABLE IN MY OWN SKIN.

Breakfast:

Snack:

Lunch:

Snack:

Dinner:

Treat:

Exercise (optional):

Think Fit™

The Stubborn Fat Gone Shake

12 raw macadamia nuts

Shrimp Caesar Salad: Toss together 5 medium cooked shrimp, 2 cups shredded romaine, 5 cherry tomatoes, and 2 Tbsp. Caesar dressing.

2 slices salami spread with cream cheese

Dijon Chicken: Pan-fry 1 chicken breast, seasoned to taste and topped with 1 Tbsp. Dijon mustard. Serve with ¼ cup sautéed zucchini, seasoned to taste.

one glass red wine (15 Sugar Calories)

Today is a rest day.

Take a moment to really let today's affirmation sink in. I want you to believe what you're saying and feel good about all the progress you've made over the past weeks. I am truly proud of your commitment and growth.

If you allow yourself to accept who you are right in this moment, you'll feel a rush of relief. That is the feeling of letting go of outward expectations and pressures, and it's also the feeling that will fuel positive action and change. Practice doing this several times a day—for just one moment at a time, allow yourself to luxuriate in complete self-acceptance.

A quote attributed to Ralph Waldo Emerson states: "To be yourself in a world that is constantly trying to make you something else is the greatest accomplishment." You are exactly who you are meant to be, so accept who you are. There is only one you, and you are unique, special, and valuable. Recognize your value, and love yourself.

Take a few minutes now to consider how your thoughts can be more accepting and loving of yourself.

> ❝ *It's not selfish to love yourself, take care of yourself, and to make your happiness a priority. It's necessary.* ❞ — Mandy Hale

HAVING A GREAT DAY COMES NATURALLY TO ME.

Breakfast:

Snack:

Lunch:

Snack:

Dinner:

Treat:

Exercise (optional):

Think Fit™

The Stubborn Fat Gone Shake

¼ cup sunflower seeds

Blue Chopped Salad: Toss together 2 cups shredded romaine, 4 slices chopped deli turkey, 1 chopped hard-boiled egg, 2 Tbsp. blue cheese crumbles, and 2 Tbsp. blue cheese dressing.

one hard-boiled egg

Grilled Flank Steak: Grill to desired doneness one 3-oz. flank steak, seasoned to taste. Serve with a side salad of 2 cups spinach, 5 sliced cherry tomatoes, 2 Tbsp. feta cheese, and a dressing of olive oil and vinegar.

one glass red wine (15 Sugar Calories)

Do a high-intensity interval training workout.

Are you happy? Scientists spend a lot of time and money studying this subject. Every other year since 1972, researchers at the University of Chicago have been questioning Americans about their attitudes and feelings in the General Social Survey, and the statistics on happiness have been surprisingly stable. Generally, one-third of Americans answer that they're "very happy," about half say that they're "pretty happy," and about 10 to 15 percent admit that they're "not too happy." Where do you fall on this spectrum?

Scientists say that happiness can be attributed to three major sources: genes, events, and values. Studies suggest that about 48 percent of how happy you feel comes from your genes, while up to 40 percent is determined by events. Well, you didn't pick your parents, you can't change your genes, and you probably don't have as much control over the path of your life as you think. So let's focus on the 12 percent of your happiness that you absolutely can affect: your values. Scientists say that the basic values of faith, family, friendships, and function are the ones that contribute most to happiness. (They actually described the last two as "community" and "work," but I'm going for alliteration here.)

Think now about these four F's: How do they impact your happiness? How can changing your actions in one area affect your state of mind?

"By choosing to be our most authentic and loving self, we leave a trail of magic everywhere we go." — Emmanuel

I **LOVE** AND **FORGIVE MYSELF** COMPLETELY.

Breakfast:

Snack:

Lunch:

Snack:

Dinner:

Treat:

Exercise (optional):

Think Fit™

The Stubborn Fat Gone Shake

12 raw macadamia nuts

Tossed Italian Salad: Toss together ½ cup steamed, chopped cauliflower; ½ cup steamed, chopped broccoli; 2 Tbsp. chopped red bell pepper; 3 sliced chopped ham; 2 Tbsp. olive oil; and salt and pepper, to taste.

2 slices salami spread with cream cheese

Cheesy Turkey Burger: Top 1 grilled turkey burger patty with 1 slice provolone, 2 slices tomato, and 1 Tbsp. mustard. Serve on ¼ cup bed of arugula.

one glass red wine (15 Sugar Calories)

Today is a rest day.

Life is a work in progress; we all make mistakes. Sometimes we lose sight of this fact, and that is okay! We weren't meant to be perfect, yet so many of us try so hard to be. "Practice makes perfect" is an expression hardwired into our brains. I say, "Let it go!" Find your inner Queen Elsa from Disney's *Frozen* and scream that from the highest mountain!

At best, practice makes *progress*. That, rather than perfection, should be your goal. Anyway, if you were actually to achieve perfection, where on earth would you go from there?

Let's all let go of the guilt of having a cheat day or eating something we probably shouldn't have. Let's not be hard on ourselves when we don't see the scale move as much as we wanted this week. Don't let these types of things be your downfall but instead your motivation to try even harder. You can do this!

Take a few minutes today to reflect on some mistakes you've made. Then remind yourself: "I forgive myself completely."

> *"What I know for sure is that there is no strength without challenge, adversity, resistance, and often pain."* — Oprah Winfrey

GREAT STRENGTH LIES WITHIN ME. I HONOR MY POWER.

Breakfast:

Snack:

Lunch:

Snack:

Dinner:

Treat:

Exercise (optional):

Think Fit™

The Stubborn Fat Gone Shake

¼ cup sunflower seeds

Shrimp Caesar Salad: Toss together 5 medium cooked shrimp, 2 cups shredded romaine, 5 cherry tomatoes, and 2 Tbsp. Caesar dressing.

one hard-boiled egg

Dijon Chicken: Pan-fry 1 chicken breast, seasoned to taste and topped with 1 Tbsp. Dijon mustard. Serve with ¼ cup sautéed zucchini, seasoned to taste.

one glass red wine (15 Sugar Calories)

Do a high-intensity interval training workout.

When you say the words of today's affirmation, you tap into your inner strength, which may be dormant from too many years of negative thinking. Affirmations bring your inner power back to life. Create your best life by honoring all that you are. Feed yourself messages that reinforce all that you deserve. Even on days when you might feel less than strong, saying that it is so will make it so.

I've included my favorite affirmations in this book because I've found such value in this practice in my own life. I say affirmations many times each day. In the morning, I like to think, *Today is going to be a great day.* If I'm feeling a little "off," I think of Émile Coué's mantra: *Every day in every way, I'm getting better and better.* Before I go to bed, I think, *Thank you, body, mind, and spirit, for giving me the strength to work hard today and strive to meet my goals.*

Harness your inner strength and don't hold back. You will feel so happy and free when you live life to its fullest. Utilize your self-confidence and surprise yourself today!

Think about a time when you were able to surprise yourself by learning or doing something new. Brainstorm more ideas of how you can stretch further in the future.

"*Just when the caterpillar thought the world was over, it became a butterfly.*" — Proverb

I AM EXACTLY WHO I WANT TO BE, AND I AM GROWING EVERY DAY.

Breakfast:

Snack:

Lunch:

Snack:

Dinner:

Treat:

Exercise (optional):

Think Fit™

The Stubborn Fat Gone Shake

12 raw macadamia nuts

Blue Chopped Salad: Toss together 2 cups shredded romaine, 4 slices chopped deli turkey, 1 chopped hard-boiled egg, 2 Tbsp. blue cheese crumbles, and 2 Tbsp. blue cheese dressing.

2 slices salami spread with cream cheese

Grilled Flank Steak: Grill to desired doneness one 3-oz. flank steak, seasoned to taste. Serve with a side salad of 2 cups spinach, 5 sliced cherry tomatoes, 2 Tbsp. feta cheese, and a dressing of olive oil and vinegar.

one glass red wine (15 Sugar Calories)

Today is a rest day.

You are transforming and changing your goals, way of eating, mind-set, and body. Like a butterfly, you're leaving behind the obstacles that once hindered you—hollow cravings, negative thoughts, and stubborn pounds. You're emerging from your cocoon light and clean, ridding yourself of more than just physical weight; negativity and lack of ambition always feel like heavy burdens. When you free yourself, you can live as you are meant to: with a full heart, happy mind, and clean body.

It takes courage to change and become a new person; but you can do it! In the past, your choices about food may have brought up feelings of shame, self-hate, or deprivation, but you can let go of them now. Those were simply learned coping mechanisms, and today you have better tools for nourishing your body and mind. Food is no longer a threat, but fuel that energizes you.

You have worked hard to release yourself from the cocoon of weight, pressures, and negativity. You are ready to fly, my friend! Let's go!

Today, contemplate all the ways in which your new life is taking flight.

"*Beauty is how you feel inside, and it reflects in your eyes. It is not something physical.*" — Sophia Loren

I AM
BEAUTIFUL
INSIDE AND OUT.

Breakfast:

Snack:

Lunch:

Snack:

Dinner:

Treat:

Exercise (optional):

Think Fit™

The Stubborn Fat Gone Shake

¼ cup sunflower seeds

Tossed Italian Salad: Toss together ½ cup steamed, chopped cauliflower; ½ cup steamed, chopped broccoli; 2 Tbsp. chopped red bell pepper; 3 sliced chopped ham; 2 Tbsp. olive oil; and salt and pepper, to taste.

one hard-boiled egg

Cheesy Turkey Burger: Top 1 grilled turkey burger patty with 1 slice provolone, 2 slices tomato, and 1 Tbsp. mustard. Serve on ¼ cup bed of arugula.

one glass red wine (15 Sugar Calories)

Today is a rest day.

Yesterday we discussed the amazing transformation of the galumphing caterpillar into the beautiful butterfly, flitting through the air. But before dismissing the caterpillar, we need to remember that all that beauty was *inside* the humble insect all along.

You are metamorphosing into something new and lovely, like the butterfly. And you are also like the *caterpillar* because you are gorgeous on the inside as well as the outside.

I find it fascinating that when someone speaks of "a beautiful person," it is the quality of inner rather than outer beauty that is usually being referred to. Of course, it is given as a tremendous compliment. What are some of the wonderful qualities inside of you that have been strengthened through your transformation these past 11 weeks? Are you kind? Generous? Thoughtful? Respectful? Loving? Take a few minutes now to think about your most beautiful qualities. Write them down, so you can remind yourself of them whenever you need to.

I encourage you to let your dreams and life take flight like the butterfly. But don't forget to stay grounded and centered like the caterpillar. No galumphing allowed, though!

17

share your celebration

You've made a commitment to change, you've stuck with it, and you're almost at the end of your Stubborn Fat Gone™ journey! But like most journeys, the end of this one is the beginning of another.

This week will be about drawing strength from the past three months and preparing yourself for your next adventure. I'll ask you to sit quietly for a bit and continue to Think Fit™. I'll also encourage you to think about how you can share the power of what you've learned with the people you care about—your friends, your family, your co-workers, and your community.

You have worked so hard to create the changes you wanted to see in yourself. Now you can be the change that you want to see in the world at large! A single person can make a dramatic difference, and that person can be you! You can inspire change in everyone around you, and your positive example can motivate the people you care about to better their lives, too.

Congratulations on making it to the end of the Stubborn Fat Gone™ program. I wish you tremendous health and happiness!

> "*All the forces in the world are not so powerful as an idea whose time has come.*"
>
> — Attributed to Victor Hugo

I AM MORE POWERFUL THAN I HAVE EVER BEEN BEFORE.

Breakfast:

Snack:

Lunch:

Snack:

Dinner:

Treat:

Exercise (optional):

Think Fit™

The Stubborn Fat Gone Shake

¼ cup pecans

Bacon Caprese Stack: Alternate 3 slices fresh mozzarella, 3 slices tomato, 3 strips cooked bacon, and 3 basil leaves in a stack. Drizzle with 1 Tbsp. balsamic vinegar.

one string cheese

Seasoned Salmon Spinach Salad: Rub one 3-oz. salmon fillet with butter and season with fresh dill. Grill, then serve atop 2 cups spinach with olive-oil-and-vinegar dressing.

one glass red wine (15 Sugar Calories)

Do a high-intensity interval training workout.

Seventy-seven days ago, you had an idea. You wanted to make powerful changes in your life, and you picked up this book. The time for your idea had come, and the effects have been profound and wide-reaching.

Today you know more than you've ever known before, which means that you hold the power to make your future even better. You have overcome so many obstacles along the way. How many times have you put down your fork, dined in rather than out, laced up your walking shoes, silenced the negative voice in your head, and cheered yourself on? Every positive change builds upon the last, and by now you have built up a wondrous amount of momentum.

I want you to honor the way that you persevere when things get tough. Because you do, you know? You are a "perseverer"! Feel the power deep inside of you. Know that you can continue to capitalize upon your success, and it will propel you to an even greater future. There's no stopping you now; you're on the move!

Take a few minutes now to think about the many obstacles you've overcome, and how you can build upon your success.

> "*If you don't love yourself, you can't love anybody else.*"
> — Jennifer Lopez

I THOROUGHLY ENJOY BEING ME.

TRACKER

Breakfast:

Snack:

Lunch:

Snack:

Dinner:

Treat:

Exercise (optional):

Think Fit™

The Stubborn Fat Gone Shake

¼ cup Brazil nuts

Crunchy Chicken Wraps: Sauté 3 oz. chopped chicken breast, 2 stalks finely chopped celery, ½ cup chopped scallions, ½ cup chopped water chestnuts, 2 Tbsp. sliced almonds, 2 Tbsp. soy sauce, and crushed red pepper to taste. Evenly divide cooked mixture between 8 romaine lettuce leaves, about 2 to 3 Tbsp. per leaf. Serve with a side of ½ cup mushrooms and 4 asparagus stalks sautéed with soy sauce.

celery sticks spread with cream cheese

Zucchini Puffs: In a bowl, mix 3 Tbsp. mayonnaise, 3 Tbsp. Parmesan cheese, 1 Tbsp. basil, and chopped garlic and lemon juice to taste. Spread mixture evenly over 2 sliced zucchini in a baking dish. Broil in oven for 1 or 2 minutes, until top is browned. Serve with a side salad of 1 cup spinach and 1 sliced tomato, dressed with lemon juice.

one glass red wine (15 Sugar Calories)

Today is a rest day.

It's one thing to feel comfortable in your own skin, but it's something entirely different to *enjoy* being yourself. That's a whole new level of satisfaction.

To enjoy yourself, you have to really *know* yourself. You've done a tremendous amount of self-reflection and soul-searching in this program already, and now you hold in your hand the tool to truly understand you!

So today I want you to schedule a date with yourself. Choose a time and place where you can be completely by yourself and enjoy your own company. Plan activities that fuel your heart, whether it's reading, knitting, or scrapbooking. Focus on the pure enjoyment of being you.

Afterward, simply sit quietly by yourself. Dedicate this time to reflecting on where you are mentally, physically, and emotionally. As you remember what you've done and appreciate the insight you've gained, think about the most valuable lesson you have learned so far.

> "*If we could change ourselves, the tendencies in the world would also change. As a man changes his own nature, so does the attitude of the world change toward him.*"
>
> — Mohandas Gandhi

I AM THE
CHANGE
I WANT TO
SEE IN THE
WORLD.

Breakfast:

Snack:

Lunch:

Snack:

Dinner:

Treat:

Exercise (optional):

Think Fit™

The Stubborn Fat Gone Shake

¼ cup pecans

Broccoli Cheese Soup: Bring 2 cups chicken broth to a simmer, add 3 cups chopped broccoli, and cook until tender. In a separate pan, gently heat 4 oz. cream cheese and ¾ cup cream on low, stirring often. Purée broccoli mixture in a blender, then blend in cream-cheese mixture. Makes 4 servings; garnish each bowl with shredded cheddar cheese.

one string cheese

Spicy Taco Salad: Sauté ¼ lb. ground beef with 1 tsp. chili powder, ½ tsp. onion powder, and 1 clove minced garlic. Add to a bowl of 2 cups chopped salad greens, 1 chopped tomato, ½ chopped bell pepper, ½ sliced avocado, 1 Tbsp. sour cream, and 2 Tbsp. chopped cilantro. Top with 2 lime wedges.

one glass red wine (15 Sugar Calories)

Do a high-intensity interval training workout.

You have accomplished something many people can't: you've changed yourself. Know that you can make a difference in other people's lives, too, in so many ways. Consider exploring one of the following websites for ideas on how:

— *Find Your Representative* (house.gov/representatives/find): The website of the U.S. House of Representatives will show you how to contact your local congressman. Encourage overhauls in the state of nutrition in this country. You can also check out the latest developments in health initiatives that will affect you and your family.

—*Alliance for a Healthier Generation* (healthiergeneration.org): The goal of this collaboration between the American Heart Association and the Clinton Foundation is to "reduce the prevalence of childhood obesity and to empower kids to develop lifelong, healthy habits." Here you will find news about the Alliance's efforts in schools and communities, along with valuable tools for raising healthy kids. President Clinton discussed with me his passion for helping improve the health of our children—his commitment to this important cause is inspiring.

— *Healthy People 2020* (healthypeople.gov): This website offers "science-based, 10-year national objectives for improving the health of all Americans." You can join the conversation on health and find links to important resources.

Now think about concrete ways you plan to contribute to the world.

> ❝*Nothing great in the world has ever been accomplished without passion.*❞
>
> — Georg Wilhelm Friedrich Hegel

I GIVE MYSELF PERMISSION TO LET MY PASSION SHINE.

Breakfast:

Snack:

Lunch:

Snack:

Dinner:

Treat:

Exercise (optional):

Think Fit™

The Stubborn Fat Gone Shake

¼ cup Brazil nuts

Bacon Caprese Stack: Alternate 3 slices fresh mozzarella, 3 slices tomato, 3 strips cooked bacon, and 3 basil leaves in a stack. Drizzle with 1 Tbsp. balsamic vinegar.

celery sticks spread with cream cheese

Seasoned Salmon Spinach Salad: Rub one 3-oz. salmon fillet with butter and season with fresh dill. Grill, then serve atop 2 cups spinach with olive-oil-and-vinegar dressing.

one glass red wine (15 Sugar Calories)

Today is a rest day.

I bet you are bursting with passion about the changes in your health and your life. That excitement is contagious! Encourage as many of your friends and loved ones to catch the "fever" of good health.

Why not invite your family to take a walk, go miniature golfing, or go bowling after dinner? You won't want to eat so much that you feel stuffed when you know you have an activity ahead of you, so it will help you stick to your plan. You'll have fun, be active, and make memories to boot.

Plan healthy outings with your friends. Rather than dishing over plates of pasta, go on a hike or bike ride. Your conversations are likely to be more stimulating and positive as you take in the sights, sounds, and smells of nature.

For your next business meeting, instead of fighting fatigue in a stuffy conference room, see if you can take the conference outside. Maybe there's a picnic table or walking trail near your office. Your meeting will be more creative because exercise gets those juices flowing. Let your best self shine!

Take a few minutes now to think of ways you can use your passion to motivate others to make healthy changes in their lives.

> "*A leader takes people where they want to go. A great leader takes people where they don't necessarily want to go, but ought to be.*"
>
> — Rosalynn Carter

I AM A LEADER, AND I INSPIRE OTHERS TO BE HEALTHIER.

Breakfast:

Snack:

Lunch:

Snack:

Dinner:

Treat:

Exercise (optional):

Think Fit™

The Stubborn Fat Gone Shake

¼ cup pecans

Crunchy Chicken Wraps: Sauté 3 oz. chopped chicken breast, 2 stalks finely chopped celery, ½ cup chopped scallions, ½ cup chopped water chestnuts, 2 Tbsp. sliced almonds, 2 Tbsp. soy sauce, and crushed red pepper to taste. Evenly divide cooked mixture between 8 romaine lettuce leaves, about 2 to 3 Tbsp. per leaf. Serve with a side of ½ cup mushrooms and 4 asparagus stalks sautéed with soy sauce.

one string cheese

Zucchini Puffs: In a bowl, mix 3 Tbsp. mayonnaise, 3 Tbsp. Parmesan cheese, 1 Tbsp. basil, and chopped garlic and lemon juice to taste. Spread mixture evenly over 2 sliced zucchini in a baking dish. Broil in oven for 1 or 2 minutes, until top is browned. Serve with a side salad of 1 cup spinach and 1 sliced tomato, dressed with lemon juice.

one glass red wine (15 Sugar Calories)

Do a high-intensity interval training workout.

Today I want you tell your friends and co-workers how excited you are about your new way of eating, moving, and thinking—that you've felt fabulous, while dropping pounds fast. Your friends won't be surprised to hear this because they've watched your incredible transformation. But I bet they would love to know your secrets so that they can become their best selves, too.

According to research, losing weight with friends, family, or co-workers leads to more long-term success. Once you share your news, you may find that some of your colleagues are interested in joining you. Just as you've had encouragement from me and your support circle, now you have the chance to be part of the support circle for someone else. What an opportunity and honor!

After you've spoken with your friends and colleagues, I want you to reflect on your experience. How did it make you feel to share with them? How did they react? And how did that make you feel?

> *"Without continual growth and progress, such words as <u>improvement</u>, <u>achievement</u>, and <u>success</u> have no meaning."* — Benjamin Franklin

I WILL CONTINUE TO CHANGE AND GROW.

Breakfast:

Snack:

Lunch:

Snack:

Dinner:

Treat:

Exercise (optional):

Think Fit™

The Stubborn Fat Gone Shake

¼ cup Brazil nuts

Broccoli Cheese Soup: Bring 2 cups chicken broth to a simmer, add 3 cups chopped broccoli, and cook until tender. In a separate pan, gently heat 4 oz. cream cheese and ¾ cup cream on low, stirring often. Purée broccoli mixture in a blender, then blend in cream-cheese mixture. Makes 4 servings; garnish each bowl with shredded cheddar cheese.

celery sticks spread with cream cheese

Spicy Taco Salad: Sauté ¼ lb. ground beef with 1 tsp. chili powder, ½ tsp. onion powder, and 1 clove minced garlic. Add to a bowl of 2 cups chopped salad greens, 1 chopped tomato, ½ chopped bell pepper, ½ sliced avocado, 1 Tbsp. sour cream, and 2 Tbsp. chopped cilantro. Top with 2 lime wedges.

one glass red wine (15 Sugar Calories)

Today is a rest day.

I believe that the key to getting rid of stubborn fat is your emotional outlook. You can't commit to a new healthy lifestyle without having the right mind-set.

By this time, I hope that you've mastered the keys to your emotional outlook. During these past 12 weeks, you've dialed down stress, anxiety, and fear, and you've dialed up happiness, contentment, and joy. You've tapped into your inner strength and wisdom. No doubt a step on the scale or a measuring tape around your waist now will prove that this journey was worth it.

As you turn the last pages of this book and end this journey, you will start another. What will that journey be?

"The future belongs to those who believe in the beauty of their dreams." — Eleanor Roosevelt

I HAVE TAKEN CHARGE OF MY HEALTH!

Breakfast:

Snack:

Lunch:

Snack:

Dinner:

Treat:

Exercise (optional):

Think Fit™

The Stubborn Fat Gone Shake

¼ cup pecans

Bacon Caprese Stack: Alternate 3 slices fresh mozzarella, 3 slices tomato, 3 strips cooked bacon, and 3 basil leaves in a stack. Drizzle with 1 Tbsp. balsamic vinegar.

one string cheese

Seasoned Salmon Spinach Salad: Rub one 3-oz. salmon fillet with butter and season with fresh dill. Grill, then serve atop 2 cups spinach with olive-oil-and-vinegar dressing.

one glass red wine (15 Sugar Calories)

Today is a rest day.

You did it! I am incredibly proud of you, and I hope that you are even more proud of yourself. Thank you for letting me walk with you on your weight-loss journey.

It is now time for you to become the mentor for yourself and perhaps even others in your life. One thing that I want you to remember as you continue with your new lifestyle is to apply the Golden Rule in reverse: Treat yourself as well as you treat others. Don't put others' needs, even those of your loved ones, so far ahead of your own that you end up neglecting your own health.

I encourage you to dream big for yourself. Perhaps it's time to plan a trip, take on a new challenge, learn a new language—the sky is the limit. Now you have the energy, happiness, and confidence to live a fulfilling life, so use this opportunity to the fullest.

Success shared is success multiplied. I would love to hear about your success! You can reach me at:

JorgeCruise.com
Facebook.com/JorgeCruise
Twitter.com/JorgeCruise

Finally, take a few minutes to reflect on how will you will be your own coach going forward.

19

frequently asked questions (FAQs)

1. Do I need to follow Think Fit™?

For you to be successful on any program you follow, you must have the mentality of success going in. If you're not fully committed to the program, what happens when any small challenges come up? You end up quitting. Think Fit™ provides you with a daily guide to help you stick to the program and give you the best chance of success.

2. Do I need to follow your eating recommendations?

Although you can lower cortisol and increase serotonin through Think Fit™ alone, following Eat Fit™ will give you the greatest advantage. It will switch your body from fat-storage mode to fat-burning mode, improve insulin resistance, and balance hormone levels. My recommendation is to follow the plan that I've laid out for you in this book, and visit JorgeCruise.com for more options.

3. Do I have to follow the menus you provided or can I follow one from your other books?

The Stubborn Fat Gone™ program is compatible with any of my other three lifestyle plans—the Belly Fat Cure™, the 100™, or Happy Hormones, Slim Belly™. Think Fit™ offers support for sticking with any healthy lifestyle. The menus in my other books are all consistent in that you will be lowering the amount of Sugar Calories you consume, while never denying yourself.

If you are unfamiliar with my other books, here's a quick rundown: Those who want rapid results should check out *The 100*™, which will help you stick with 100 Sugar Calories per day or less. Women over 40, especially those concerned with menopause, should read *Happy Hormones, Slim Belly*™, which will show you the powerful effects of Carb Cycling (alternating between 2 days at 100 Sugar Calories and 5 days at 500 Sugar Calories) on your hormone levels, mood, and weight loss. And my *Belly Fat Cure*™ series for carb lovers offers another way of looking at and tracking sugar, with dozens of recipes, menu planners, and more.

4. Can I drink alcohol?

Yes, you can still enjoy adult beverages in moderation. I suggest a glass of wine in the evening, two at the most. However, if you find that you're not losing weight on this program, I recommend avoiding alcohol.

5. How can I reduce more of my stress levels?

Beyond following the Think Fit™ recommendations mentioned, there are a few other things you can do:

— *Deep breathing.* Take five minutes to focus on your breath, inhaling through your nose and exhaling through your mouth. This will provide a boost of oxygen to your body and allow your mind to decompress from any stress you've been going through. (You may also want to review Dr. Weil's breathing exercise from Day 54.)

— *Meditation, or taking time for yourself.* A moment of self-reflection or just getting some "me time" can be the ticket. Think about how you felt the last time you got that opportunity . . . can you even remember when you were able to do so? Maybe now is the time to take a mini-vacation, visit the nail salon, or go to a movie. Often we are so busy helping others that we forget to help ourselves.

— *Enjoying the moment.* Have you ever been riding in a car, on a route you've driven hundreds of times before, and as you looked out the widow you thought, *Wow, I never noticed that before*? We get too caught up with daily activities to stop and smell the roses, so to speak. At the very least, as you're going about your usual day, look up and take notice of the sky. Upon reflection, the blueness of it and the gentle pace of the clouds can be amazing.

6. How can you be my coach beyond the book?

I've had the privilege of helping people in their homes, via e-mail, on the phone, and recently on Facebook in a private group. Through my experiences, I've learned that going digital is the best way for me to help on a scale that makes sense for my availability and is cost-effective for my clients. If you are interested in my digital coaching program, with videos and *live* support, please visit StubbornFatGone.com for the complete package that can take you to the next level.

7. How do I get more variety in meals?

There are three easy ways of getting more variety:

1. Use the food lists in this book or look at nutrition labels to come up with meals that allow you to stick under your daily Sugar Calorie limit.

2. Purchase *The 100*™, *Happy Hormones, Slim Belly*™, or any of the titles in my *Belly Fat Cure*™ series. All of these books contain dozens of healthy recipes, all of which are low in sugar, to help you stay under your allotment.

3. The easiest method is to go to JorgeCruise.com and join for free. You'll get more meal planners, recipes, and food lists in digital format, which makes planning simple.

8. How quickly will I see changes?

My clients tell me that they notice results almost immediately. Within the first two days, both weight loss and a sense of renewal will come to you. A large number of my clients experience significant weight loss after the first week, especially those who have more than 30 pounds to lose. Those with 15 to 20 pounds to lose tend to experience a 2- to 5-pound weight loss that first week, but some lose up to 9.

While it all depends on your commitment and the amount you have to lose, I promise you this: Stick to the Stubborn Fat Gone™ plan as I have outlined, and you'll see dramatic results!

9. Will this plan work for my whole family?

Yes, Stubborn Fat Gone™ is a healthy lifestyle for everyone in your family. Positive thoughts, exercise, and monitoring Sugar Calories are all important to overall health for children, teens, adults, and seniors, regardless of gender or body weight.

10. How can I share with you about the weight I've lost?

I'm always eager to hear about the success my clients have on this program. I encourage you to share your story, along with before and after photos, on my Facebook page: Facebook.com/JorgeCruise.

11. What products or supplements should I consider for best results?

I am a fan of simplicity, so this program is designed to be sustainable without any specialty products or supplements. However, I do have some shortcuts I recommend: specifically the Stubborn Fat Gone Shake and fiber blend. These breakthrough products help you stay on track in the morning and are everything your body needs for breakfast. When I make a Stubborn Fat Gone Shake, I can run around and feel amazing until lunchtime.

For my favorite shortcut products and recommendations, please read the next section and visit JorgeCruise.com/Resources to see what may be right for you.

health resources

The following are my recommended supplements for additional weight loss, hormonal balance, stress relief, and other great benefits. To purchase any of these health resources and aid your specific goals, please visit JorgeCruise.com/Resources.

Carb Control: Dietary Enzymes

Carb Control is designed to help reduce the digestion of starches and absorption of glucose while improving the digestion of protein-containing foods. This can help those who have a difficult time controlling their carbohydrate intake and are in need of blood-glucose control, which can lead to greater success with healthy weight management.

Carb Control features a non-GMO form of a common white bean (*Phaseolus vulgaris*), a proprietary amylase inhibitor. It also has green coffee extract (GCE), which contains chlorogenic acid, which is shown to assist with weight management and body composition through its support of proper glucose absorption in the gut and triglyceride levels in the liver.

CLA: Natural Fat-Melting Enhancer

Conjugated linoleic acid (CLA) is a naturally occurring fatty acid shown to be useful in supporting proper fat burning and healthy blood-sugar levels as well as in modulating inflammation. CLA also has strong antioxidant properties.

Insulin Control: Chromium Caps

Insulin Control is a synergistic formula of nutrients for optimal insulin function and blood-sugar control. It combines the best chelated minerals from Albion Advanced Nutrition in a base of cinnamon powder to assist insulin receptor function and cellular glucose uptake.

Flawless Skin: Natural GLA softgels

Flawless Skin softgels supply gamma linolenic acid from the oil of borage seeds. GLA is essential for smooth and healthy skin and female hormonal balance.

Superior Creatine: Load-Free 900 mg Creatine Monohydrate

With Superior Creatine, which contains an impressive 900 mg of buffered creatine monohydrate per capsule, only one or two capsules per day are required. Many of the unpleasant side effects of high-dose creatine supplementation (e.g., nausea, diarrhea, cramps, and bloating) are not from the creatine, but from the waste metabolite creatinine. Since Superior Creatine is the only creatine with a pH above 12, it will not convert to creatinine in liquids such as the bloodstream. This results in less of the aforementioned side effects and more creatine delivered to the muscle and other tissues. This means better results at much lower doses (no more "loading") when compared with regular creatine powder.

Omega Lemon Smoothie: High-Potency Fish Oil

Each 2-teaspoon serving is packed with 1,100 mg of EPA and 720 mg DHA for a total of 1,820 mg of omega-3 fatty acids. It is manufactured using a proprietary emulsification technology that significantly reduces the size of fish-oil molecules, resulting in enhanced absorption. This formula is ideal for children and those who do not prefer to swallow softgels.

Essential Fiber: Wild Berry–Flavored and Unflavored

As a dietary supplement, take 5 grams (approximately 2 teaspoons) per day. I recommend that you take it with the Jorge Cruise Protein Shakes to feel satiated all morning. Consume extra water when taking Essential Fiber.

Having enough fiber is one of the secrets to weight loss and a healthy gut. Essential Fiber contains 12 different types of fiber to replicate naturally occurring fiber in the diet, and it reduces appetite by helping you feel full while slowing down your blood-sugar response to keep insulin at healthy levels. Essential Fiber also helps you absorb nutrients better.

Green Machine: Lemon Lime–Flavored and Unflavored Greens

Getting your vegetable count in each day is a whole lot easier with Green Machine. Alkalizing nutrient-dense vegetables contain the highest source of vitamins, minerals, prebiotics, enzymes, and antioxidants without sugar and processed carbs. As a dietary supplement, mix 9 grams (approximately 1 tablespoon) in water per day.

Mito Support: Anti-aging and Energy Support

Mito Support is designed to help support optimal mitochondrial biogenesis, which is critical for the promotion of healthy aging, optimal energy production, and protection from reactive oxygen species (oxidative stress).

Mito Support features pyrroloquinoline quinone (PQQ), a water-soluble, vitamin-like compound, and *Rhodiola rosea,* a popular adaptogen. PQQ is an enzyme cofactor that possesses antioxidative, neuroprotective, and cardioprotective properties that encourage mitochondrial biogenesis. *Rhodiola rosea* helps support the adrenal glands. Research shows that *Rhodiola rosea* is a powerful herb for enhancing mitochondrial energy production, and it helps defend against free radicals in the nervous system as well as the mitochondria.

Stress Proof: Natural Stress Fighter

Stress Proof is a uniquely formulated product that provides gamma-aminobutyric acid (GABA), a key neurotransmitter in the body involved in a normal calm stress response. It also supplies other calming nutrients, including glycine, niacinamide, pantothenic acid, and vitamin B_6.

Collagen Support: Lemon-Flavored MSM Powder

Collagen Support powder contains the sulfur-supplying compound methylsulfonylmethane (MSM), which modulates histamine release and inflammation. It also has the ability to support collagen production, which is the primary constituent of cartilage, skin, and connective tissue.

B-12 Lozenges: High-Dose Vitamin B-12

Vitamin B_{12} lozenges are a great-tasting, high-dose vitamin B_{12} product. Each berry-flavored lozenge contains 5,000 mcg methylcobalamin, the activated form of vitamin B_{12}. They are designed to deliver B_{12} through the mucous membranes in order to bypass the need for intrinsic factor, a protein produced in the stomach that is needed for maximal gastrointestinal absorption of B_{12}.

Liquid Sunshine: Vitamin D and K Immune Support

This formula contains high therapeutic doses of vitamin D_3 and vitamin K (as both K_1 form and MK_7, a form of K_2) for situations where more aggressive repletion is required. Vitamins D and K are essential for optimal bone and arterial health and for maintaining the immune system in proper balance. The amount of vitamin D and K in this formula may be beneficial for those who do not get adequate sun exposure and/or dietary sources of these vitamins. As these two vitamins work as a team, increasing doses of vitamin D will increase the need for vitamin K.

Jorge Cruise Protein Shake: Iced Vanilla Latte or Chocolate

As a dietary supplement, mix 27 grams (approximately one scoop) in 8 ounces of water or any unsweetened beverage. It pairs well with the Essential Fiber for a morning shake that will curb hunger and give you good nutrients to help you feel energized all morning.

For many, whey protein shakes can cause gas, bloating, skin irritation, congestion, and even weight gain, because whey shakes have the tendency to cause insulin spikes, which leads to fat storage.

This new source of protein is derived from hormone-free, GMO-free, free-range beef from Sweden called HydroBEEF. You get all the benefits of whey but none of the negative side effects. Also unique to this product is the amount of naturally occurring, complete collagen proteins that promote connective tissue.

The best part of this protein is the taste. Milky smooth and pleasant to drink every morning or during the day. Mixes easily with a shaker bottle or blender, or stirred with a spoon.

Max Energy: High-Fiber Coconut Energy Bar

Consume one bar at a time, anytime you are hungry or need natural energy. It is considered a Freebie food under any of the Jorge Cruise plans.

Energy Boost: Medium-Chain Triglycerides

As a dietary supplement, take 11 grams (approximately 2 teaspoons) with a meal or with a Jorge Cruise Protein Shake. Energy Boost is an excellent source of medium-chain triglycerides (MCTs) from coconut and palm oil, and is mainly comprised of two fatty acids that are quickly and easily absorbed, giving you a readily available source of energy.

Probiotic+: 15 Billion Probiotic Cultures

Probiotic+ treats the cause of constipation, dysbacteriosis. It helps increase essential vitamins, including B_{12} and K, while regulating inflammation and immune-system responses, as well as protecting against inflammatory diseases. Probiotic+ ensures the survival of the bacteria through three major barriers: the manufacturing process, the store shelf, and your stomach acid. Probiotic+ has a patented delivery system that is designed to ensure the highest potency of the live organisms delivered to your intestinal tract.

Complete Multivitamin

Complete Multivitamin is a full-spectrum multivitamin with Albion chelated minerals for maximum absorption and bioavailability. This powerhouse multivitamin supplies supportive nutrients not normally found in regular multivitamins, such as alpha lipoic acid, TMG, fruit bioflavanoids, choline, and inositol. This formula also contains high gamma tocopherol (vitamin E); high levels of all the B vitamins, including the proprietary NatureFolate™ blend of active isomer naturally occurring folates; and natural mixed carotenoids.

Essential Enzymes

Essential Enzymes contain a combination of enzymes that are capable of aiding digestion. Betaine HCL and the enzyme pepsin both aid in the digestion of protein. This formula also contains special proteolytic enzymes as well as amylase, invertase, and lactase to further aid in the digestion of starch, lactose (milk sugar), protein, and fat. As a dietary supplement, take one capsule per day with a meal.

Melatonin Sleep: 3 mg

As a dietary supplement, adults can take one tablet per day, 20 minutes before bedtime, for a great night's sleep.

selected bibliography

Abbott, Elizabeth. 2008. *Sugar: A Bittersweet History.* London and New York: Duckworth Overlook.

American Psychological Association. 2012, January 11. "Stress in America: Our Health at Risk." Retrieved from www.apa.org/news/press/releases/stress/2011/final-2011.pdf.

Anson, MR. 2003. "Intermittent fasting dissociates beneficial effects of dietary restriction on glucose metabolism and neuronal resistance to injury from calorie intake." *Proceedings of the National Academy of Sciences of the United States of America.* 100(10): 6216–20.

Aubrey, A. 2006, November 16. "Teaching kids the science of calories." National Public Radio. Retrieved from www.npr.org/templates/story/story.php?storyId=6493713.

Avena, NM, et al. 2008. "Evidence for sugar addiction: Behavioral and neurochemical effects of intermittent, excessive sugar intake." *Neuroscience and Biobehavioral Reviews.* 32(1):20–39.

Banting, W. 1869. *Letter on Corpulence, Addressed to the Public.* 4th edition. London: Harrison. Retrieved from www.lowcarb.ca/corpulence/index.html.

Berk, LS, et al. 2008. "Cortisol and Catecholamine stress hormone decrease is associated with the behavior of perceptual anticipation of mirthful laughter." *The FASEB Journal.* 22 (1): 946.11.

Bhathena, SJ, et al. 1991. "Effects of omega 3 fatty acids and vitamin E on hormones involved in carbohydrate and lipid metabolism in men." *Am. J. Clin. Nutr.* 54(4): 684–8.

Bichsel, SE. 1988. "An overview of the U.S. beet sugar industry." *Chemistry and processing of sugarbeet and sugarcane,* eds. MA Clarke and MA Godshall.

Brehm, BJ, et al. 2003. "A Randomized Trial Comparing a Very Low Carbohydrate Diet and a Calorie-Restricted Low Fat Diet on Body Weight and Cardiovascular Risk Factors in Healthy Women." *The Journal of Clinical Endocrinology & Metabolism.* 88(4): 1617–23.

Brillat-Savarin, JA. 1986. *The Physiology of Taste.* Translated by MF Fisher. San Francisco: North Point Press.

Brummett, BH, et al. 2012. "Cortisol responses to emotional stress in men: association with a functional polymorphism in the 5HTR2C gene." *Biol Psychol.* Jan 89(1): 94–8.

Cagnacci, A, et al. 1997. "Melatonin enhances cortisol levels in aged women: reversible by estrogens." *J. Pineal Res.* 22(2): 81–5.

Cahill, GF, et al. 1959. "Effects of insulin on adipose tissue." *Annals of the New York Academy of Sciences.* Sept 25(82):4303–11.

Carney, DR, et al. 2010. "Power posing: brief nonverbal displays affect neuroendocrine levels and risk tolerance." *Psychol Sci.* Sept 21 (10): 1363–68.

Clear, James. "How Long Does It Actually Take to Form a New Habit? (Backed by Science)." The Huffington Post. Retrieved from www.huffingtonpost.com/jame-clear/forming-new -habits_b_5104807.html.

Cloud, J. 2009, August 9. "Why exercise won't make you thin." *Time* magazine. Retrieved from www.time.com/time/printout/0,8816,1914974,00.html.

Cohn, V. 1980, August 31. "A passion to keep fit: 100 million Americans exercising." *The Washington Post.*

Cordain L, et al. 2000. "Plant-animal subsistence ratios and macronutrient energy estimations in worldwide hunter-gatherer diets." *American Journal of Clinical Nutrition.* 71(3): 682–92.

Correll, J, et al. 2004. "An affirmed self and an open mind: Self-affirmation and sensitivity to argument strength." *Journal of Experimental Social Psychology,* 40: 350–6.

Creswell, J, et al. 2013. "Self-Affirmation Improves Problem-Solving under Stress." *PLoS ONE.* 8(5): e62593.

Dancel, JF. 1864. *Obesity, or Excessive Corpulence: The Various Causes and the Rational Means of Cure.* Translated by Barrett, M. Toronto: W.C. Chewett.

Delarue J, et al. 2003. "Fish oil prevents the adrenal activation elicited by mental stress in healthy men." *Diabetes Metab.* 29(3): 289–95.

Diamond, D. 2011, May 20. "How Bad Science and Big Business Created the Obesity Epidemic." University of South Florida, College of Arts and Sciences. Retrieved from www.youtube.com/watch?v=3vr-c8GeT34.

Dietler, Michael, and Brian Hayden, eds. 2001. *Feasts: Archaeological and Ethnographic Perspectives on Food, Politics, and Power.* Washington, D.C.: Smithsonian Institution Press.

Donaldson, BF. 1962. *Strong Medicine.* Garden City, NY: Doubleday.

Ebbeling, CB, et al. 2012. "Effects of dietary composition on energy expenditure during weight-loss maintenance." *Journal of the American Medical Association.* 307(24): 2627–34.

Epel, ES, et al. 2000. "Stress and body shape; stress-induced cortisol secretion is consistently greater among women with central fat." *Psychosomatic Medicine.* Sep–Oct 62(5): 623–32.

Fichter, MM, et al. 1986. "Weight loss causes neuroendocrine disturbances: experimental study in healthy starving subjects." *Psychiatry Res* 17(1): 61–72.

Field, et al. 2005. "Cortisol decreases and serotonin and dopamine increase following massage therapy." *Int. J. Neurosci.* 115(10): 1397–413.

Fogelholm, M, et al. 2000. "Does physical activity prevent weight gain—a systematic review." *Obesity Reviews.* 1(2): 95–111.

Fulkerson, WJ, and BY Tang. 1979. "Ultradian and circadian rhythms in the plasma concentration of cortisol in sheep." *J. Endocrinol.* 81(1): 135–41.

Gleeson, M. 2006. "Can nutrition limit exercise-induced immunodepression?" *Nutr. Rev.* 64(3): 119–31.

Golf, SW, et al. 1998. "On the significance of magnesium in extreme physical stress." *Cardiovasc Drugs Ther.* 12 Suppl 2: 197–202.

Groesz, L, et al. 2012. "What is eating you? Stress and the drive to eat." *Appetite.* 58(2): 717–21.

Haas, VK, et al. 2009. "Body composition changes in female adolescents with anorexia nervosa." *Am. J. Clin. Nutr.* 89(4): 1005–10.

Haist, RE, and CH Best. 1966. "Carbohydrate Metabolism and Insulin." *The Physiological Basis of Medical Practice,* 8th edition, eds. CH Best and NM Taylor. Baltimore: Williams & Wilkins.

Hargrove, JL. 2006. "History of the calorie in nutrition." *The Journal of Nutrition.* 136: 2957–61.

Harvey, W. 1872. *On Corpulence in Relation to Disease: With Some Remarks on Diet.* London: Henry Renshaw.

Harvie, MN, et al. 2011. "The effects of intermittent or continuous energy restriction on weight loss and metabolic disease risk markers: a randomized trial in young overweight women." *International Journal of Obesity.* 35(5): 714–27.

Hellhammer, J, et al. 2004. "Effects of soy lecithin phosphatidic acid and phosphatidylserine complex (PAS) on the endocrine and psychological responses to mental stress." *Stress.* 7(2): 119–26.

Higginson, J. 1997. "From Geographical Pathology to Environmental Caricnogenesis: A Historical Reminiscence." *Cancer Letters.* 117: 133–42.

Hoffman, FL. 1937. *Cancer and Diet.* Baltimore: Williams & Wilkins.

Howard, JM. 2012. *The History of the Pancreas.* The Pancreas Club: Los Angeles, CA. Retrieved from http://pancreasclub.com/home/pancreas.

Husband, AJ, et al. 1973. "The effect of corticosteroid on absorption and endogenous production of immunoglobulins in calves." *Aust J Exp Biol Med Sci.* 51(5): 707–10.

Indiana University. 2010. "Obesity, Type 2 Diabetes, and Fructose." Office of Science Outreach; Dept. of Biology. The Trustees of Indiana University. Retrieved from www.indiana.edu/~oso/Fructose/Consequences.html.

Jaremka, LM. 2011. "Reducing defensive distancing: Self-affirmation and risk regulation in response to relationship threats." *Journal of Experimental Social Psychology.* 47: 264–8.

Johnson, RK, et al. 2009. "Dietary Sugars Intake and Cardiovascular Health: A Scientific Statement From the American Heart Association." *Circulation.* Retrieved from http://circ.ahajournals.org/content/120/11/1011.full.pdf.

Josse, R. "Nibbling versus Gorging: Metabolic Advantages of Increased Meal Frequency." *New England Journal of Medicine*: 929–34.

Kennedy, ET, et al. 2001. "Popular Diets: Correlation to health, nutrition, and obesity." *Journal of the American Dietetic Association.* April 101(4): 411–20.

Keys, A. 1980. *Seven Countries: A Multivariate Analysis of Death and Coronary Heart Disease.* Cambridge, MA: Harvard University Press.

Keys, A, et al. 1950. *The Biology of Human Starvation*, Vols. I–II. Minneapolis, MN: University of Minnesota Press.

Kipple, KF, and KC Ornelas. 2000. *The Cambridge World History of Food.* Cambridge University Press. Retrieved from www.cambridge.org/us/books/kiple/sugar.htm.

Kotwica, G, et al. 2002. "Effects of mating stimuli and oxytocin on plasma cortisol concentration in gilts." *Reprod Biol.* 2(1): 25–37.

Kraemer, WJ, et al. 2009. "Recovery from a national collegiate athletic association division I football game: muscle damage and hormonal status." *J Strength Cond Res.* 23(1): 2–10.

Kraus, WE. "Effects of aerobic vs. resistance training on visceral and liver fat stores, liver enzymes, and insulin resistance by HOMA in overweight adults from STRRIDE AT/RT." *AJP: Endocrinology and Metabolism:* E1033–39.

Lally, P, et al. 2010 "How are habits formed: Modelling habit formation in the real world." *European Journal of Social Psychology.* Oct: Vol 40(6): 998–1009.

Larsson, SC, et al. 2006. "Consumption of sugar and sugar-sweetened foods and the risk of pancreatic cancer in a prospective study." *American Journal of Clinical Nutrition.* 84(5): 1171–6.

Lefcourt, AM, et al. 1993. "Circadian and ultradian rhythms of peripheral cortisol concentrations in lactating dairy cows." *J. Dairy Sci.* 76(9): 2607–12.

Legault, L, et al. 2012. "Preserving Integrity in the Face of Performance Threat: Self-Affirmation Enhances Neurophysiological Responsiveness to Errors." *Psychological Science.*

Leibel, RL, et al. 1995. "Changes in energy expenditure resulting from altered body weight." *New England Journal of Medicine.* 332(10): 621–8.

Leproult, R, et al. 1997. "Sleep loss results in an elevation of cortisol levels the next evening." *Sleep.* 20(10): 865–70.

Lewis, GF, et al. 2002. "Disordered fat storage and mobilization in the pathogenesis of insulin resistance and type 2 diabetes." *Endocrine Reviews.* 23(2): 201–9. Retrieved from http://edrv .endojournals.org/content/23/2/201.full.pdf+html.

Lovallo, WR, et al. 2006."Cortisol responses to mental stress, exercise, and meals following caffeine intake in men and women." *Pharmacol. Biochem. Behav.* 83(3): 441–7.

Maglione-Garves, CA, et al. "Stress Cortisol Connection: Tips on Managing Stress and Weight." University of New Mexico. Retrieved from www.unm.edu/~lkravitz/Article%20folder/stresscortisol.html.

Malik, VS, and FB Hu. 2012. "Sweeteners and Risk of Obesity and Type 2 Diabetes: The Role of Sugar-Sweetened Beverages." *Current Diabetes Reports* 12(2): 195–203.

Maratos-Flier, E, and JS Flier. 2005. "Obesity." *Joslin's Diabetes Mellitus.* 533–45.

Marketdata Enterprises, Inc. 2014. "The U.S. Weight Loss Market: 2014 Status Report & Forecast." Retrieved from www.marketresearch.com/Marketdata-Enterprises-Inc-v416/Weight-Loss-Status-Forecast-8016030.

Moberg, GP, and JA Mench. 2000. *The Biology of Animal Stress: Basic Principles and Implications for Animal Welfare.* Wallingford, Oxon, UK: CABI Pub.

Moyer, AE, et al. 1994. "Stress-induced cortisol response and fat distribution in women." *Obesity Research.* May; 2(3): 255–62.

Moyer, MW. 2010, "Carbs against cardio: More evidence that refined carbohydrates, not fats, threaten the heart." *Scientific American.* Retrieved from www.scientificamerican.com/article.cfm?id=carbs-against-cardio.

Newburgh, LH. 1930. "The Nature of Obesity." *Journal of Clinical Investigation.* 8(2): 197–213.

———. 1948. "Energy Metabolism in Obese Patients." *Bulletin of the New York Academy of Medicine.* 24(4): 227–38.

O'Connell, J, and K Hawkes. 1981. "Alyawara Plant Use and Optimal Foraging Theory." *Hunter-Gatherer Foraging Straegies,* eds. B Winterhalder and E Smith. Chicago: University of Chicago Press.

Pennington, AW. 1953. "Treatment of Obesity with Calorie Unrestricted Diets." *American Journal of Clinical Nutrition.* 1(5): 343–8.

Pirozzo, S, et al. 2002. "Advice on low-fat diets for obesity." *Cochrane Database System Review.* (2):CD003640.

Quiroga, MC, et al. 2009. "Emotional and Neurohumoral Responses to Dancing Tango Argentino: The Effects of Music and Partner." *Music and Medicine.* 1(1): 14–21.

Reaven, GM. 1988. "Banting lecture 1988. Role of insulin resistance in human disease." *Diabetes.* 37: 1595–607.

Robson, PJ, et al. 1999. "Effects of exercise intensity, duration and recovery on in vitro neutrophil function in male athletes." *Int J Sports Med.* 20(2): 128–35.

Roiser, JP, et al. 2008. "The Effect of Acute Tryptophan Depletion on the Neural Correlates of Emotional Processing in Healthy Volunteers." *Neuropsychopharmacology.* 33: 1992–2006.

Samaha, FF, et al. 2003. "A Low-Carbohydrate as Compared with a Low-Fat Diet in Severe Obesity." *The New England Journal of Medicine.* 348: 2074–81.

Sanchez, A, et al. 1973. "Role of sugars in human neutrophilic phagocytosis." *The American Journal of Clinical Nutrition.* 26(11): 1180–4.

Sandle, GI, et al. 1981. "The effect of hydrocortisone on the transport of water, sodium, and glucose in the jejunum. Perfusion studies in normal subjects and patients with coeliac disease." *Scand. J. Gastroenterol.* 16(5): 667–71.

Schernhammer, ES, et al. 2005. "Sugar-Sweetened Soft Drink Consumption and Risk of Pancreatic Cancer in Two Prospective Cohorts." *Cancer Epidemiology, Biomarkers & Prevention.* 14(9): 2098–105.

Schulze, MB, et al. 2004. "Sugar-sweetened beverages, weight gain, and incidence of type 2 diabetes in young and middle-aged women." *Journal of the American Medical Association.* Aug 25; 292(8): 927–34.

Shalev, I, et al. 2009. "BDNF Val66Met polymorphism is associated with HPA axis reactivity to psychological stress characterized by genotype and gender interactions." *Psychoneuroendocrinology.* 34(3): 382–8.

Sharot, T, et al. 2007. "Neural mechanisms mediating optimism bias." *Nature.* Nov 1; 450(7166): 102–5.

Sher, L. 2005. "Type D Personality: the heart, stress, and cortisol." *QJM: An International Journal of Medicine*, 98(5): 323–9.

Sherman, DK, and GL Cohen. 2006. "The psychology of self-defense: Self-affirmation theory." *Advances in Experimental Social Psychology,* Vol 38, ed. MP Zanna. San Diego, CA: Academic Press.

Silverman, Marni N, et al. "Immune Modulation of the Hypothalamic-Pituitary-Adrenal (HPA) Axis during Viral Infection." *Viral Immunology.* 18(1): 41–78.

Smith, JL, et al. 2009. *Advanced nutrition and humanmetabolism.* Belmont, CA: Wadsworth Cengage Learning.

Speth, J, and K Spielmann. 1983. "Energy Source, Protein Metabolism, and Hunter-Gatherer Subsistence Strategies." *Journal of Anthropological Archaeology.*

Starks, MA, et al. 2008. "The effects of phosphatidylserine on endocrine response to moderate intensity exercise." *J Int Soc Sports Nutr.* 5:11.

Steptoe, A, et al. 2007. "The effects of tea on psychophysiological stress responsivity and post-stress recovery: a randomised double-blind trial." *Psychopharmacology.* 190(1): 81–9.

Stimson, RH, et al. 2009. "Cortisol release from adipose tissue by 11beta-hydroxysteroid dehydrogenase type 1 in humans." *Diabetes.* 58(1): 46–53.

Tappy, L, and E Jéquier. 1993. "Fructose and dietary thermogenesis." *American Journal of Clinical Nutrition.* Nov 58(5 supplement): S766–70.

Taubes, Gary. 2007. *Good Calories, Bad Calories: Fats, Carbs, and the Controversial Science of Diet and Health.* New York: Anchor Books.

——. 2011. *Why We Get Fat: And What to Do About It.* New York: Anchor Books.

——. 2011, February 17. "Is Sugar Toxic?" *The New York Times.* Retrieved from www.nytimes.com/2011/04/17/magazine/mag-17Sugar-t.html.

Trapp, EG, et al. 2008. "The effects of high-intensity intermittent exercise training on fat loss and fasting insulin levels of young women." *International Journal of Obesity.* 32(4): 684–91.

Uedo, N, et al. 2004. "Reduction in salivary cortisol level by music therapy during colonoscopic examination." *Hepatogastroenterology.* 51(56): 451–3.

Verboeket-van de, WP, and KR Westerterp. 1993. "Frequency of feeding, weight reduction and energy metabolism." *International Journal of Obesity and Related Metabolic Disorders.* 17(1): 31–6.

Weerth de, C, et al. 2003, August. "Development of cortisol circadian rhythm in infancy." *Early Hum. Dev.* 73(1–2): 39–52.

Wilborn, CD, et al. 2004. "Effects of Zinc Magnesium Aspartate (ZMA) Supplementation on Training Adaptations and Markers of Anabolism and Catabolism." *J Int Soc Sports Nutr.* 1(2): 12–20.

Williams, WR. 1908. *The Natural History of Cancer with Special Reference to Its Causation and Prevention.* London: William Heinemann.

Wood, J, et al. 2009. "Positive Self-Statements: Power for Some, Peril for Others." *Psychological Science.* 20(7): 860–6.

Young, CM, et al. 1953. "Reducing and Post-Reducing Maintenance on the Moderate Fat Diet: Metabolic Studies." *Journal of the American Dietetic Association.* 29(9): 890–6.

acknowledgments

A big thank-you to the amazing Hay House team: Alex Freemon, Stacey Smith, Margarete Nielsen, Charles McStravick, Lindsay McGinty, Patricia Lopez, Tiffini Alberto, Heather Tate, Wioleta Gramek—and, most especially, to my dear friend Reid Tracy for taking on this project and sharing my vision. Thank you for your immense belief in this project and your work to impact people's lives on a global scale. Also, I would like to thank a very special woman—Louise Hay—for her commitment to bringing a wealth of desperately needed information to the world. Your commitment and passion deserve a standing ovation.

I owe particular gratitude to my amazing team, as without them, nothing would be possible. To Kristin Penne, for keeping us all organized, on time, and sane. Your support and assistance means so much. To Oliver Stephenson, I could not have done it without your direction and support. You truly know how to apply your incredible commitment and talent to our mission. You make it all run! To Leslie Marcus, for your incredible insights and wisdom, you are amazing. And to Jennifer Reich, without your hard work this book would not exist.

I am so grateful to have met JJ Virgin and to call her my friend. You embody a wonderful community of support for the greater good. Thank you for your years of support on questioning the conventional dieting and fitness wisdom and thinking for yourself.

A very special thank-you to my invaluable circle of experts: Gary Taubes, Dr. Robert Lustig, Dr. Mehmet Oz, Dr. Nicholas Perricone, Dr. Christiane Northrup, Dr. David Ludwig, and Michael Pollan. And to Dr. Andrew Weil, thank you for your constant support and feedback.

To my clients—your support in helping me refine this program, offering your comments, tips, and the courage to change your own lives have been a gift—thank you. You all inspire me each and every day.

I wish to thank so many others who have contributed to this book as well as my overall vision and mission. Their advice, knowledge, and support have been so valuable and I would not be where I am today without them. While the list could go on and on, I wish to thank a few of them here, in alphabetical order.

THANK YOU

Abra Potkin	Bobbi Brown
Al Roker	Bobby Flay
Alexandra Cohen	Bruce Barlean
Andreas Koch	Carol Brooks
Andy Jenkins	Cathy Chermol
Andy McNicol	Daniel Sheldon
Anthony Robbins	David Tompson
Art Smith	Diane Sawyer
Beth Robb	Dustin Nigilo
Bill Clinton	Eben Pagan
Bill Geddie	Edward Ash-Milby
Bob Wietrak	Emeril Lagasse

Evan Dollard

Frank Kern

Ginnie Roeglin

Hanna Richert

Heath Squier

Hilary Estey
    McLoughlin

Howard Bragman

Jacqui Stafford

Jairek Robbins

Janet Annino

Jay Robb

Jessica Ortner

Jessica Scosta

Joanna Parides

Joe Fusco

John Redmann

Jon Davidson

Jonathan Lizoette

Jose Pretlow

Joseph Quesada

Katie Couric

Kelly Ripa

Lance Bass & the Dirty
    Pop Team
    @ SiriusXM Satellite
    Radio

Linda Fennell

Lindsey Pfeiler

Lisa Gregorisch-
    Dempsey

Maggie Jaqua

Marc Victor

Mario Batali

Mark Sisson

Marta Fox

Martha Stewart

Mary Amicucci

Mary Ellen Keating

Mel Maurer

Michael Koenings

Michelle McGowen

Natalie Morales

Nick Ortner

Niki Vettel

Oprah Winfrey

Pennie Ianniciello

Rachael Ray

Richard Galanti

Richard Heller

Robin Meade

Robin Roberts

Sage Robbins

Scott Eason

Stephen Steigler

Steve Harvey

Sushupti Yalamanchili

Suzanne Somers

Suze Orman

Terence Noonan

Tim Austgen

Tim Mantoani

Tim Talevich

Tod Jones

Toni Richi

Wayne Dyer

Jorge Cruise
about the author

JORGE CRUISE is the #1 *New York Times* best-selling fitness author of over 20 diet and fitness books in over 16 languages. He is a contributor to *The Dr. Oz Show, Steve Harvey, Good Morning America,* the *Today* show, the *Rachael Ray Show, EXTRA TV, Huffington Post, First for Women Magazine,* and the *Costco Connection.*

Connect with Jorge socially at:

Facebook.com/JorgeCruise

YouTube.com/JorgeCruise

JorgeCruise.Tumblr.com

Instagram.com/JorgeCruise

Twitter.com/JorgeCruise

Pinterest.com/JorgeCruise

Plus.Google.com/+JorgeCruisePlus

We hope you enjoyed this Hay House book.
If you'd like to receive our online catalog featuring additional information on
Hay House books and products, or if you'd like to find out more about
the Hay Foundation, please contact:

Hay House, Inc., P.O. Box 5100, Carlsbad, CA 92018-5100
(760) 431-7695 or (800) 654-5126
(760) 431-6948 (fax) or (800) 650-5115 (fax)
www.hayhouse.com® • www.hayfoundation.org

Published and distributed in Australia by:
Hay House Australia Pty. Ltd., 18/36 Ralph St., Alexandria NSW 2015
Phone: 612-9669-4299 • *Fax:* 612-9669-4144 • www.hayhouse.com.au

Published and distributed in the United Kingdom by:
Hay House UK, Ltd., Astley House, 33 Notting Hill Gate, London W11 3JQ
Phone: 44-20-3675-2450 • *Fax:* 44-20-3675-2451 • www.hayhouse.co.uk

Published and distributed in the Republic of South Africa by:
Hay House SA (Pty), Ltd., P.O. Box 990, Witkoppen 2068
Phone/Fax: 27-11-467-8904 • www.hayhouse.co.za

Published in India by:
Hay House Publishers India, Muskaan Complex, Plot No. 3, B-2, Vasant Kunj, New Delhi 110 070
Phone: 91-11-4176-1620 • *Fax:* 91-11-4176-1630 • www.hayhouse.co.in

Distributed in Canada by:
Raincoast Books, 2440 Viking Way, Richmond, B.C. V6V 1N2
Phone: 1-800-663-5714 • *Fax:* 1-800-565-3770 • www.raincoast.com

Take Your Soul on a Vacation

Visit www.HealYourLife.com® to regroup, recharge, and reconnect
with your own magnificence. Featuring blogs, mind-body-spirit news,
and life-changing wisdom from Louise Hay and friends.

Visit www.HealYourLife.com today!

Join for FREE

Go to JorgeCruise.com to try your first week for *FREE*

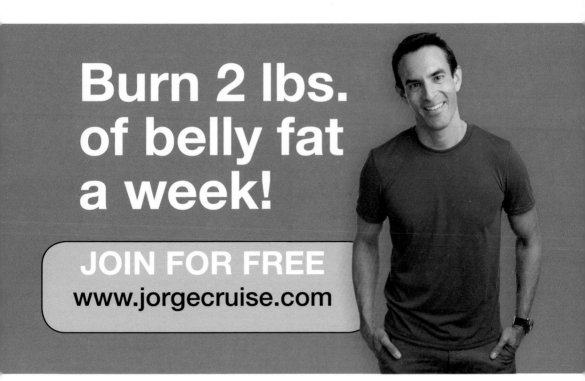

Burn 2 lbs. of belly fat a week!

JOIN FOR FREE
www.jorgecruise.com

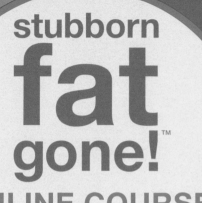

stubborn fat gone!™

ONLINE COURSE

with Jorge Cruise

For even more in-depth information, videos, recipes, examples, and coaching, reserve your space for the **Stubborn Fat Gone Online Course!**

Discover how to drop the fat that bothers you most with Jorge's personal coaching videos plus printable menus and more digital resources to help you stay on track!

Offering "anywhere" support from your laptop, tablet, or smartphone, Jorge provides coaching via private Facebook group, motivational videos, and access to information while you're out and about. Imagine standing in line at Starbucks and having the information you need at your fingertips!

Eat your favorite foods, overcome obstacles, and keep off the fat! Take information from the book a step further and make these easy lifestyle changes permanent.

FIND OUT MORE AT

www.hayhouse.com/stubborn-fat-gone-course